AF743999

Antisense Therapy

Edited by Shashwat Sharad and Suman Kapur

Published in London, United Kingdom

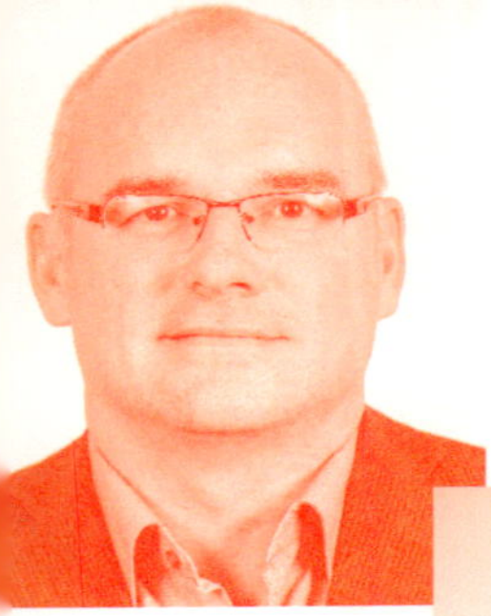
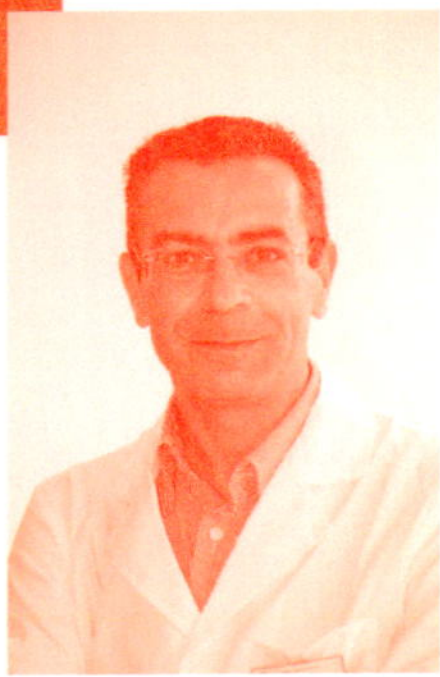
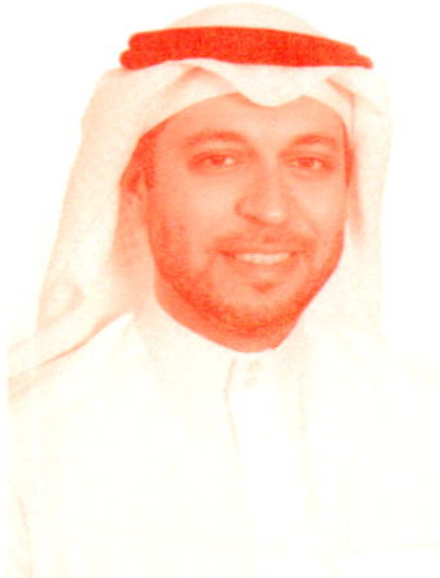
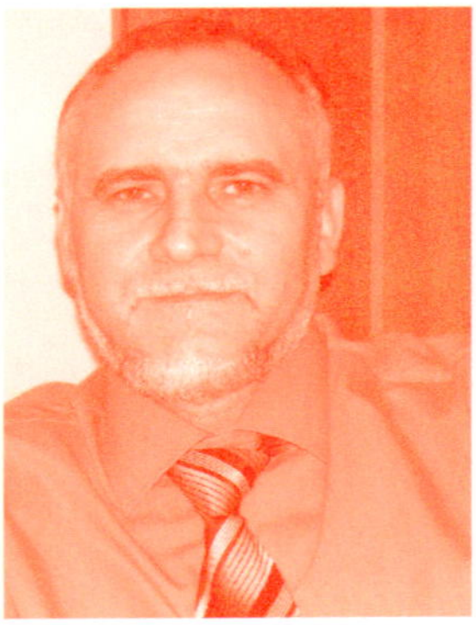
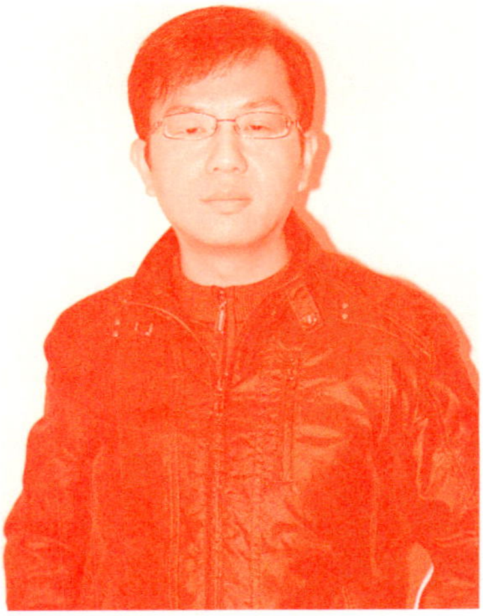
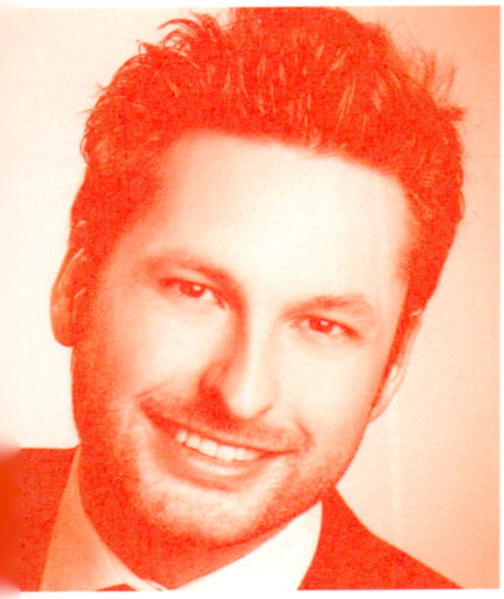
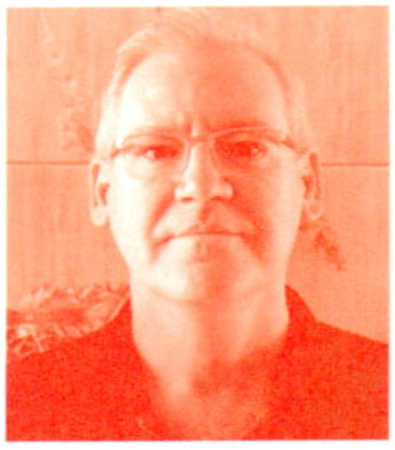

IntechOpen

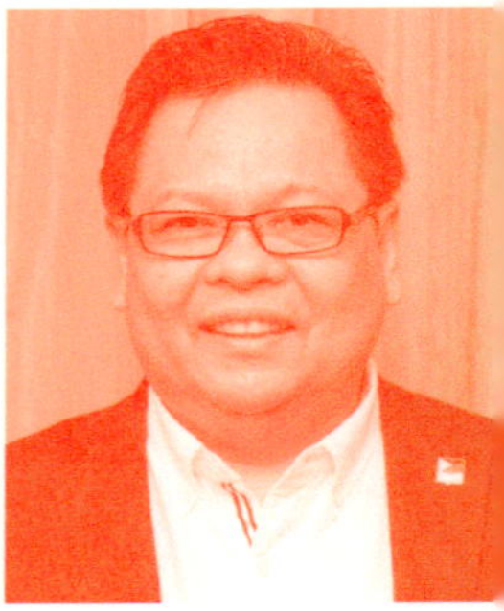
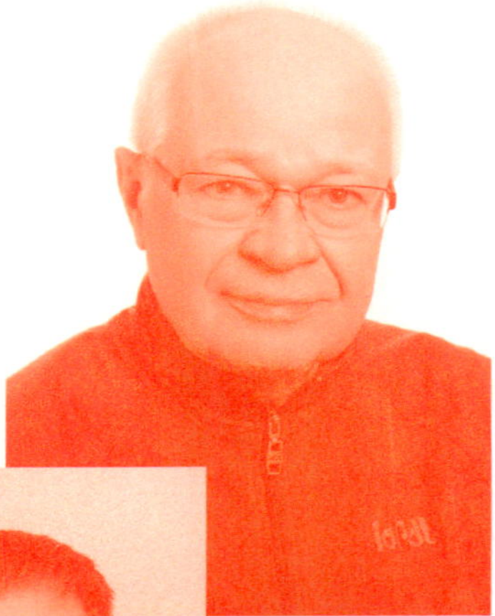
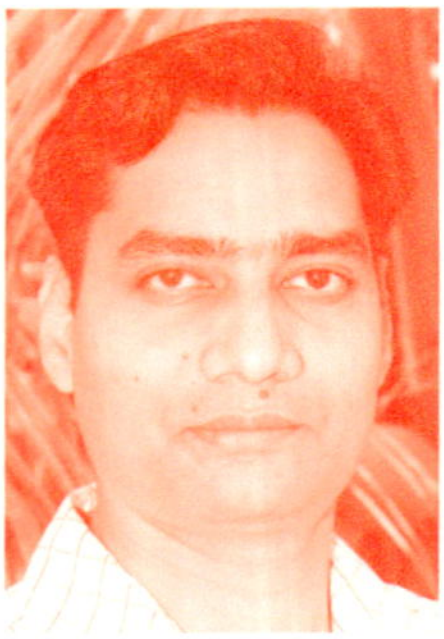
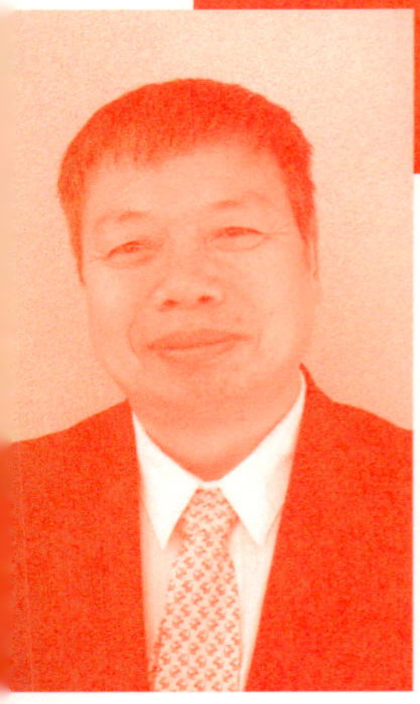
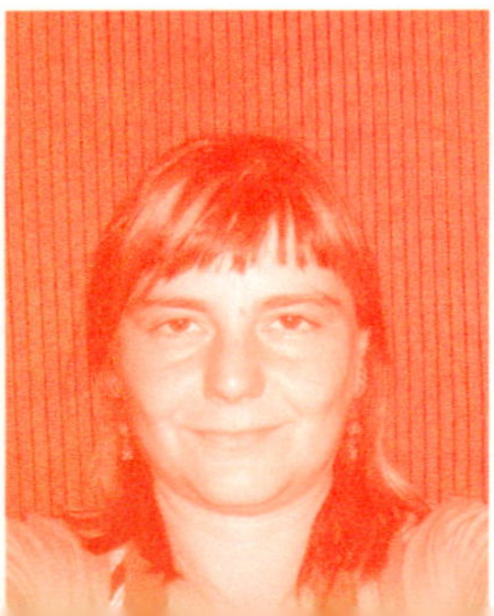
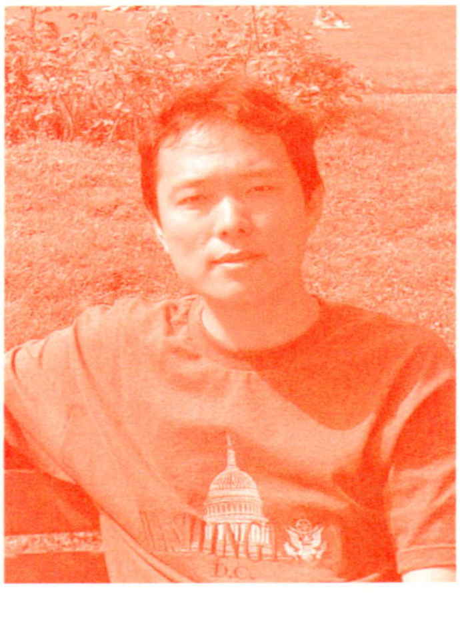

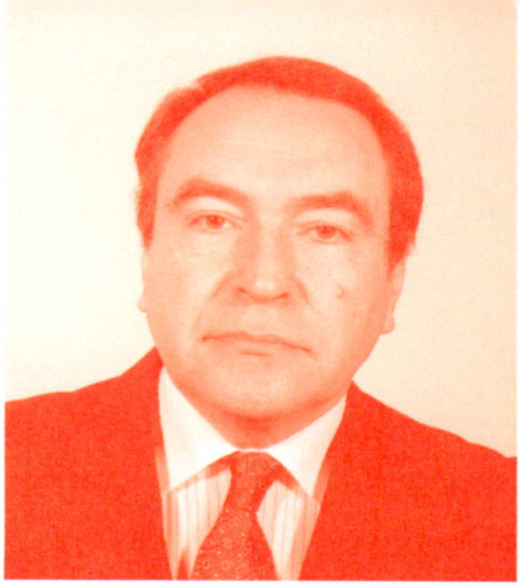

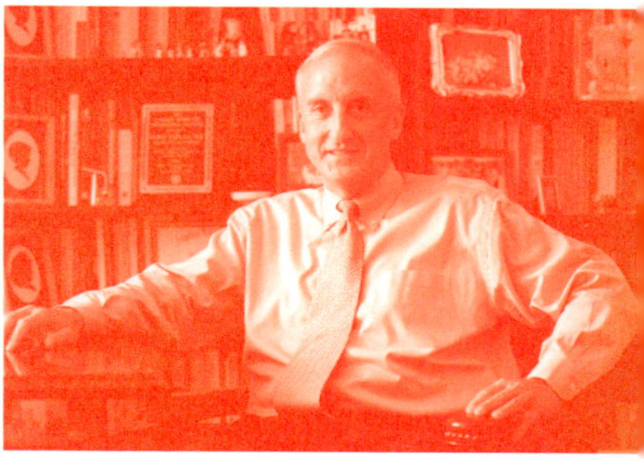

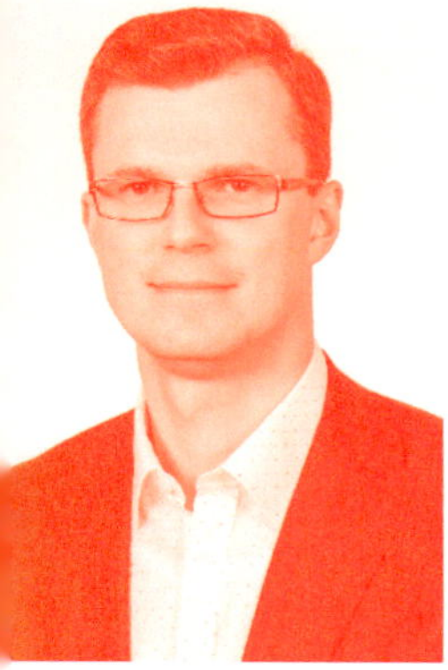

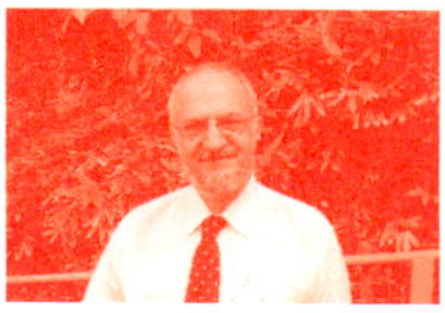

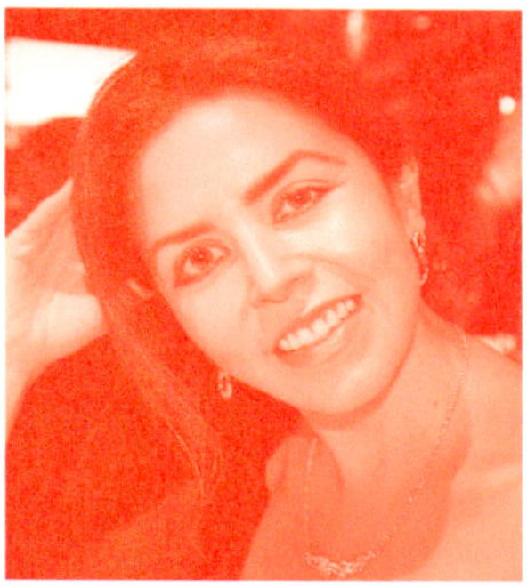

Supporting open minds since 2005

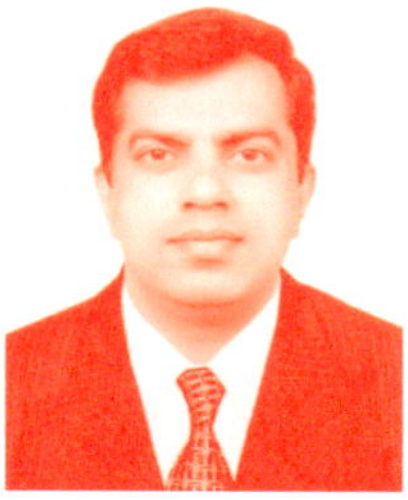

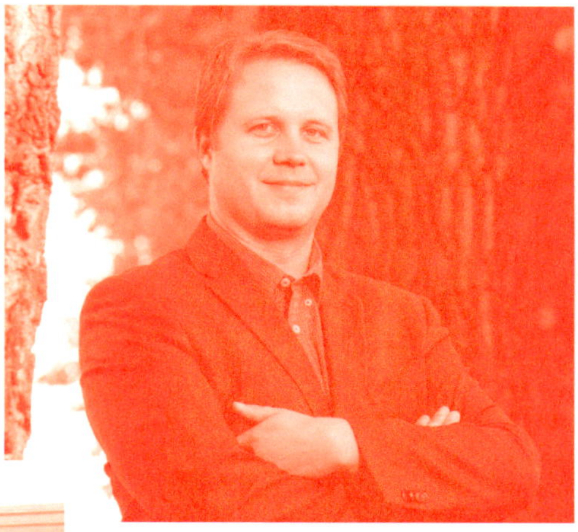

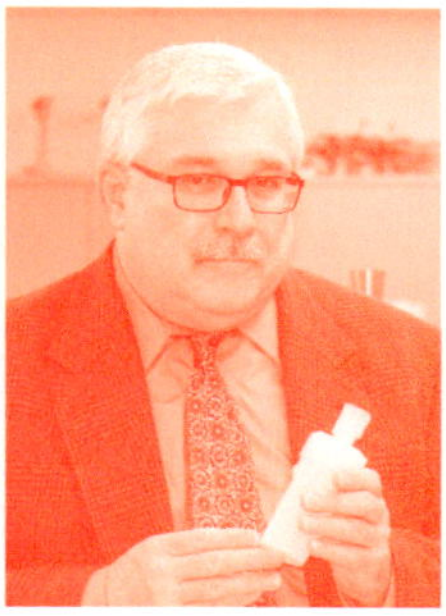

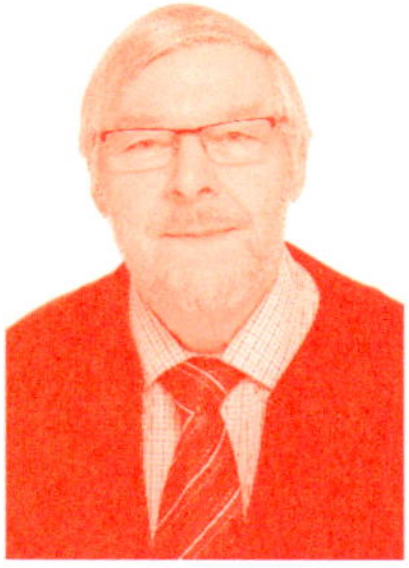

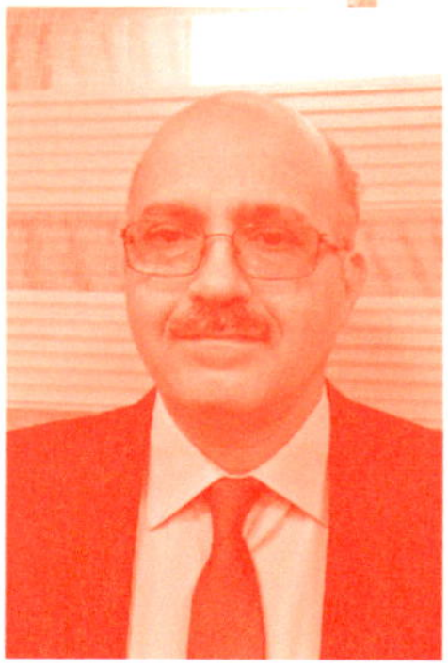

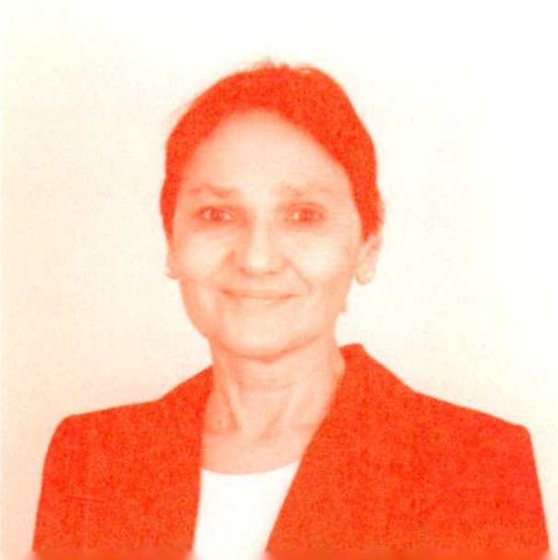

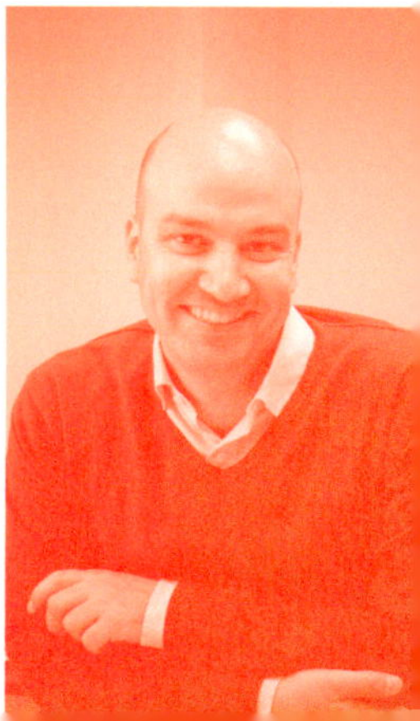

Antisense Therapy
http://dx.doi.org/10.5772/intechopen.73736
Edited by Shashwat Sharad and Suman Kapur

Contributors
Behiye Şenel, Gülay Büyükköroğlu, Ovidiu Balacescu, Oana Baldasici, Simona Visan, Loreadana Balacescu, Catalin Vlad, Patriciu Achimas, Andrew Walayat, DaLiao Xiao, Meizi Yang, Jerzy Trojan, Palma Rocchi, Sara Karaki, Clement Paris, Shashwat Sharad

© The Editor(s) and the Author(s) 2019
The rights of the editor(s) and the author(s) have been asserted in accordance with the Copyright, Designs and Patents Act 1988. All rights to the book as a whole are reserved by INTECHOPEN LIMITED. The book as a whole (compilation) cannot be reproduced, distributed or used for commercial or non-commercial purposes without INTECHOPEN LIMITED's written permission. Enquiries concerning the use of the book should be directed to INTECHOPEN LIMITED rights and permissions department (permissions@intechopen.com).
Violations are liable to prosecution under the governing Copyright Law.

(cc) BY

Individual chapters of this publication are distributed under the terms of the Creative Commons Attribution 3.0 Unported License which permits commercial use, distribution and reproduction of the individual chapters, provided the original author(s) and source publication are appropriately acknowledged. If so indicated, certain images may not be included under the Creative Commons license. In such cases users will need to obtain permission from the license holder to reproduce the material. More details and guidelines concerning content reuse and adaptation can be found at http://www.intechopen.com/copyright-policy.html.

Notice
Statements and opinions expressed in the chapters are these of the individual contributors and not necessarily those of the editors or publisher. No responsibility is accepted for the accuracy of information contained in the published chapters. The publisher assumes no responsibility for any damage or injury to persons or property arising out of the use of any materials, instructions, methods or ideas contained in the book.

First published in London, United Kingdom, 2019 by IntechOpen
IntechOpen is the global imprint of INTECHOPEN LIMITED, registered in England and Wales, registration number: 11086078, 7th floor, 10 Lower Thames Street, London, EC3R 6AF, United Kingdom
Printed in Croatia

British Library Cataloguing-in-Publication Data
A catalogue record for this book is available from the British Library

Additional hard and PDF copies can be obtained from orders@intechopen.com

Antisense Therapy
Edited by Shashwat Sharad and Suman Kapur
p. cm.
Print ISBN 978-1-78984-532-7
Online ISBN 978-1-78984-533-4
eBook (PDF) ISBN 978-1-78985-265-3

For EU product safety concerns:
IN TECH d.o.o., Prolaz Marije Krucifikse Kozulić 3, 51000 Rijeka, Croatia, info@intechopen.com or visit our website at intechopen.com.

We are IntechOpen, the world's leading publisher of Open Access books

Built by scientists, for scientists

4,400+
Open access books available

117,000+
International authors and editors

130M+
Downloads

151
Countries delivered to

Our authors are among the
Top 1%
most cited scientists

12.2%
Contributors from top 500 universities

CLARIVATE ANALYTICS
BOOK CITATION INDEX
INDEXED

WEB OF SCIENCE™

Selection of our books indexed in the Book Citation Index in Web of Science™ Core Collection (BKCI)

Interested in publishing with us?
Contact book.department@intechopen.com

Numbers displayed above are based on latest data collected.
For more information visit www.intechopen.com

Meet the editors

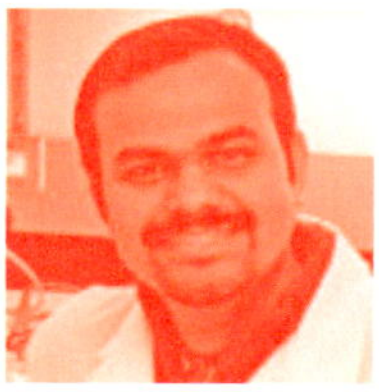

Dr. Shashwat Sharad is Assistant Professor and Staff Scientist at the Center for Prostate Disease Research, Uniformed Services University–Walter Reed Surgery, USA. He is a member of the John P. Murtha Cancer Center at Walter Reed. For decades, he dedicated his research efforts to addressing molecular genetic alterations in prostate cancer with emphasis on translating new information for the benefit of patients. His current research focuses on (1) defining prostate cancer-specific gene and protein alterations and hormonal mechanisms through evaluations of prostate cancer genome, transcriptome and proteome and cancer biology approaches; and (2) developing/evaluating new technologies for improving diagnosis, prognosis and treatment of prostate cancer. He played a key role in the successful outcome of a multidisciplinary translational research effort between urologists, cancer biologists, pathologists, epidemiologists, and bio and medical informaticians. This synergy has been highlighted by several publications. Dr. Sharad is a biomedical translational researcher with a strong academic/administrative track record. He is the recipient of several research fellowships and grant awards. He has published various manuscripts, review articles, book chapters and conference proceedings. Several students, fellows and residents trained by him have gone on to make excellent careers for themselves. He actively serves as an editorial board member and reviewer for leading journals. He made a great impact on science by contributing to developing the technology for the point-of-care device, RightBiotic: The Fastest Antibiotic Finder.

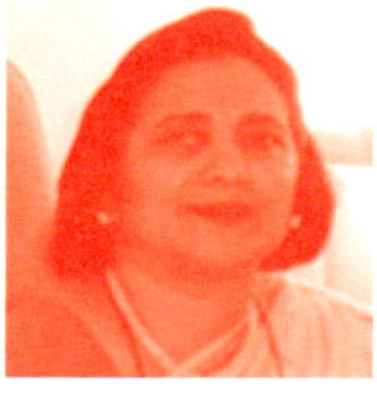

Dr. Suman Kapur is Senior Professor and Dean at the Birla Institute of Technology and Science (BITS) Pilani, Hyderabad Campus. Her research interests include genetic markers for vulnerability to chronic human diseases, screening strategies for low-cost settings, medical devices for field deployment in low-resource settings, and disease prevention through natural products. Dr. Kapur has received several awards and has been honored by Government of India as a Women Achiever in the field of Science and Technology. She holds several patents, has published and/or edited several books, has published more than 200 peer-reviewed scientific articles, has delivered more than 220 invited/keynote lectures, and has organized several scientific meetings, workshops, and dedicated trainings. Dr. Kapur is also an entrepreneur and has a startup that strives to provide affordable healthcare for all. She is the recipient of several awards including the Marico Foundation "Innovate for India Award," the Ricoh Education Foundation "Innovation Ninja Award," and a Photon Research Award for her work in antimicrobials. She is an expert member on several panels related to stem cell therapeutics, functional foods and nutraceuticals (FSSAI), standards for food and water requirements during disaster management (NDMA), and jury member for several award committees for awards in science.

Contents

Preface

Antisense therapy, or oligotherapy, is an emerging field of disease treatment and a revolution that has completely changed gene therapy. Antisense oligonucleotides are small synthetic fragments of DNA that have potential to target and bind to messenger RNA of a particular gene causing a particular disease, and modulate specific protein production in human genome. Antisense therapy using oligonucleotides has many applications in clinical medicine and has great potential to change the therapeutic landscape for many disease conditions, including their prevention, treatment, and management. This book presents oligonucleotides as an important therapeutic option and discusses how they may be used to treat cancer and other diseases. It not only covers important developments in the field of molecular mechanisms, but also highlights novel therapeutic approaches in several human disorders including cancer. There was a need to bring this information together in a single volume, as much of the recent developments are dispersed throughout biomedical literature, largely in specialized journals.

It is my hope that readers will appreciate the complexity of oligonucleotides research, especially for healthcare treatment. In the era of precession medicine, targeted therapy plays an important role. Identifying disease-specific molecular changes and targets for precision treatment is critical. In theory, oligonucleotides are designed to control the transfer of genetic information, but the use of antisense therapy is likely to benefit the patient and help manage disease. This book summarizes the current state of the field of oligo-based therapy in cancer and is an ideal resource for clinicians and researchers interested in antisense therapy. It will also appeal to physicians, surgeons, residents, biomedical scientists, and students.

Shashwat Sharad, Ph.D.
Center for Prostate Disease Research,
Department of Surgery,
Uniformed Services University of Health Sciences (USU) and
Walter Reed National Military Medical Center (WRNMMC),
Bethesda, Maryland, USA

Henry Jackson Foundation for the Advancement of Military Medicine,
Bethesda, Maryland, USA

Suman Kapur, Ph.D.
Senior Professor,
Department of Biological Sciences and Dean,
International Programmes and Collaboration Division (University wide),
Birla Institute of Technology and Science,
Pilani Hyderabad Campus, Telangana, India

Chapter 1

Antisense Therapy: An Overview

Shashwat Sharad

Abstract

Nucleic acids are the backbone of antisense therapy. Antisense oligonucleotide-based therapeutics involves downregulation of gene expression. RNA-based drugs that include antisense oligonucleotides bear great therapeutic potential toward treatment of various diseases by altering RNA and/or reducing, restoring, and modifying protein expression through multiple molecular mechanisms. Pharmacology of targeted antisense therapy has provided the platform to translate its utility to the clinic. Over the years, chemical modifications of antisense oligonucleotides have not only enhanced the specificity and efficacy but also reduced the side effects. These have changed the whole clinical trial design and provide newer strategies for therapies. Improvement in antisense oligonucleotide therapy technology has allowed and brought research from bench to clinic. Additionally, the use of small interfering RNAs, micro RNAs, ribozymes, and other antisense compounds toward the treatment of deadly diseases like cancers have demonstrated both preclinical and clinical responses. Furthermore, antisense therapy has great potential to target specific genes of interest in the context of precision medicine. Optimization of enhanced delivery, specificity, affinity, and nuclease resistance with reduced toxicity is underway in different disease context. This chapter gives a complete overview of antisense therapy and highlights its potential. Here, we focused on the advances of the antisense technology, pharmacology, therapeutics, and drug discovery.

Keywords: antisense oligonucleotides, antisense therapy, antisense drug, antisense therapeutic, gene therapy

1. Introduction: antisense technology

The advancement in the next-generation sequencing enables us to identify the genetic heritages of several diseases, such as cancer, Parkinson's, rheumatoid arthritis, and Alzheimer's, which brings to attention the development of personalized medicine [1]. This knowledge has been well adapted and accepted for diagnosis, but the field still lags toward pharmaceutical interventions to address the genetic defects underlying diseases. At present, small molecules and proteins are the two major classes of US Food and Drug Administration (FDA)-approved drugs [2]. Small-molecule drugs inhibit target proteins through competitive binding, whereas protein-based drugs (such as antibodies) can bind with high specificity to several targets. The size and stability of proteins are the major limitations of their utility for majority of disease targets [2], and both protein and small-molecule drugs cannot target every disease-relevant protein or gene. Thus, there is a current need to develop the drugs for personalized genomics. The mRNA- and DNA-based drugs are therapeutically more promising and have the great potential to cure the genetic defect [1]. The RNA-based drugs have emerged as a promising candidate to treat

IntechOpen

diseases at the genetic (gene and RNA) levels. The delivery of therapeutic RNA has been limited due to several numbers of factors such as nucleic acid design, delivery methods, and materials for transport of RNA drugs to the site of interest [1]. The current advancement in RNA and RNA-protein therapy has shown the great potential for the development of RNA delivery, and the clinical applications of RNA-based drugs have been proven by modulating gene/protein expression and gene editing [1].

An approach to fight disease by utilizing short DNA-like molecules is known as antisense oligonucleotides. This is the most effective and commonly used technology to regulate the gene expression and drugs for targeted gene therapy. These antisense oligonucleotides bind to messenger RNA (mRNA) and impair the protein production and inhibit the gene expression. The antisense molecules are synthetic replica of specific mRNA sequence to block the function of the specific target gene of interest in the human genome. Recently, antisense therapy has emerged as a promising tool to treat various diseases, and for treatment, several antisense drugs have been approved by the FDA. For antisense gene therapy, chemically engineered oligonucleotides complementary to specific mRNA are inserted into the cells which stop the translation of the specific protein. Similarly, the antisense drug contains the vital molecule—"the noncoding mRNA"—which blocks the translation of a specific protein. The antisense oligonucleotides could be very useful to treat the viral diseases, genetic/hereditary diseases, as well as cancers. The naturally occurring oligonucleotides bear poor stability and very low specificity and have a lot of side effects in vivo. The therapeutic use of oligonucleotides can be achieved by enhancing the stability and specificity of the molecules and reducing the side effects by chemical modification. The most common therapeutic oligonucleotides are small interfering RNA, ribozyme, DNAzyme, anti-gene, CpG, decoy, and aptamer. The chemical modification of antisense oligonucleotides can improve their ability to enter the cells to bind the specific target gene sequences which further disrupt the targeted gene function. Several antisense RNA and antisense oligonucleotide delivery systems such as virus vectors (retrovirus, adenovirus, and adeno-associated virus) and liposomes have been developed to carry the antisense RNA or oligonucleotides through the cell membrane into the cytoplasm and nucleus. The oligonucleotides mainly target the ribonucleic acid (RNA), whereas small molecules and antibodies primarily target proteins due to their chemical properties and distinct molecular mechanism of action. The mRNA codes for protein to noncoding RNAs (such as microRNA, transfer RNA, small interfering RNAs, ribosomal RNA, and long noncoding RNAs). The main function of noncoding RNAs is the transfer of genetic information from DNA to protein [3]. The major therapeutic approach to target RNA-based therapy is antisense oligonucleotides because of their high affinity, selectivity, ease of chemical modifications, and less toxicity. This chapter will provide a comprehensive overview of antisense therapy and their major therapeutic approaches.

The remarkable progress in the field of gene therapy and antisense therapy is apparent from numerous gene therapy- and antisense therapy-based clinical trials that are currently underway worldwide.

Gendicine (Ad-p53), the first gene therapy-based product, was approved in China for the treatment of head and neck squamous cell carcinoma in conjunction with radiotherapy. One AON drug, Vitravene, had been also approved for the local treatment of cytomegalovirus-induced retinitis, and several others are in clinical trials, including those siRNAs, miRNAs, and ribozymes that are targeting the mRNA of different oncogenes and other cancer-promoting genes.

Although the application of gene therapy and antisense therapy to mediate tumor regression is well demonstrated in experimental and clinical settings, impediment remains when translating this into large clinical application. The main obstacles that remained in cancer gene therapy and antisense therapy are the lack of delivery systems that successfully deliver an efficacious dose of a therapeutic gene (s) or antisense drug(s) to the targeted tumor site. Targeted gene or antisense drug delivery to distant tumors for therapeutic approaches is a demanding task that urges the development of delivery vectors capable of overcoming many barriers. Many scientists have used viral and non-viral vectors to deliver the therapeutic gene or antisense compound in to the targeted tumor cells or tissues. Although the results of early gene therapy- and antisense therapy-based clinical trials using either viral or non-viral vectors have been encouraging, still it is difficult to find a single method that meets all the conditions for an ideal gene transfer and vector expression.

Limitations of the present vector technologies have slowed the progress of gene therapy and antisense therapy for cancer to the clinic. Thus, the development of appropriate delivery systems for targeting therapeutic genes and antisense agents into targeted tumor cells and tissues is one of the potential approaches that have to be further explored in the future in order to augment gene therapy and antisense therapy against a wide range of cancers. It is hoped that the next generation of carriers could be a promising technology for systemic cancer gene therapy and antisense therapy.

2. Pharmacology of antisense drugs

The antisense oligonucleotides have the potential to manipulate the gene expression which prompted the field toward the therapeutic application and value of oligonucleotides as potential drugs and their targets [4]. The direct route to target RNA in a selective way is a well-established platform for drug discovery. The well-defined mechanisms, uncomplicated and easy to design, bring antisense oligonucleotides as a promising candidate for therapeutic development. The therapeutic potential of antisense drugs for the treatment of several diseases is already translated from bench to bedside, and many antisense drugs have entered into clinical trials for the treatment. The first patent on antisense therapy was granted to Molecular Biosystems company in 1991 for developing the antisense compounds. The first FDA-approved antisense product drug was afovirsen developed by Ionis Pharmaceuticals in 1992 which was a phosphorothioate oligonucleotide that targeted mRNA sequence of the E2 gene, which is associated with human papillomavirus transcription and replication. Later oblimersen, a phosphorothioate oligonucleotide, was designed to target the Bcl-2 protein for the treatment of melanoma and certain leukemias. Unfortunately, both the drugs failed in the clinical trial programs due to lack of efficacy and failure to demonstrate overall survival benefits and dose-limiting toxicity. Currently, several gene therapy- and antisense therapy-based clinical trials are ongoing. The major challenge of antisense drugs is effective and safe delivery to the target. The advancement toward antisense-based drug delivery is in progress. Several chemical modifications, novel chemistries, better formulation, and design of oligonucleotide not only have improved the potency and tolerability of antisense drug but also have enhanced the drug distribution to the targeted RNA inside the cells [5, 6]. The clinical application of antisense drugs requires safe and efficient carrier system, and currently, the viral and non-viral vectors are the most common methods used to deliver the antisense drugs specifically to the target tissues and cells. The viral vector-based delivery is most advantageous due to their high transfection efficiency [7]. Also, the new chemistries and better antisense oligonucleotide designs further improve the unwanted side effects, safety, and tolerability. From the last three decades, several antisense drugs have entered into clinical trials and market for the treatment of a broad variety of diseases, and numerous oligonucleotides are under clinical development [6, 8–10]. The first-generation antisense drug, fomivirsen, targeting cytomegalovirus, was approved for the treatment of cytomegalovirus retinitis [11]. Many second-generation drugs are under development and are showing encouraging activity in the clinic. Now oligonucleotide therapy has come a long way and has been established as promising therapeutic tool. During this period, several clinical trials have been performed on thousands of participants for several diseases and only six molecules provided the clear clinical benefit in rigorously controlled trials [10]. As of now, there are six FDA-approved drugs based on oligonucleotide therapy: (1) fomivirsen for treatment of CMV retinitis in AIDS patients, (2) mipomersen for treatment of familial hypercholesterolemia, (3) defibrotide for treatment of veno-occlusive disease in the liver, (4) eteplirsen for the treatment of Duchenne muscular dystrophy, (5) pegaptanib for the treatment of neovascular age-related macular degeneration, and (6) nusinersen for the management of spinal muscular atrophy [10, 12]. In conclusion oligonucleotide-based antisense therapy has provided solutions to untreatable diseases. Future inventions in this technology will help in establishing the better and affordable cure to many more diseases.

3. Antisense therapeutic interventions in various diseases

The antisense technology is well placed to influence the developments in human genetics and genomics to generate drugs for the treatment of monogenic and polygenic diseases. The "antisense" are the oligodeoxyribonucleotide molecules complementary to the DNA or RNA sequence of the target gene designed to hybridize specific mRNA. By capitalizing "antisense" DNA approach, the overexpressed proteins can be blocked in several diseases such as cancer, neurological diseases, cardiovascular diseases, inflammation and autoimmune diseases, infectious diseases, etc. [6].

3.1 Antisense therapy for cancer

The beauty of antisense technology is that it can precisely recognize the DNA location in a gene, a single mRNA class, and can distinguish between the normal and mutated oncogenes in cancer cells. Several studies have confirmed that in cancer patients, this can be used as an inhibitor of gene expression, which will decrease the tumor growth by manipulating the important cellular functions and protein production. By decreasing the specific gene expression, inducing the degradation of target mRNA, and initiating the premature termination of transcription, the antisense therapy can correct the abnormal expression of cellular genes and mutations in tumor cells. One of the major limitations of this approach is nuclease degradation. For this, several strategies are under development. Delivery of antisense oligo or drug to distant as well target tumors is a major hurdle. The development of suitable delivery systems for targeting therapeutic genes and antisense agents into targeted tumor cells and tissues is one of the potential approaches that needs to be further developed and explored. In order to enhance the gene therapy and antisense therapy against a wide variety of cancers and cancer types in future, the development of next generation of carriers will a remarkable progress in the field of gene therapy and could serve as a promising technology for systemic cancer gene therapy and antisense therapy. As we know, cancer has been a major area of therapeutic investigation for antisense technology. Currently, custirsen, a chimeric 2′MOE-modified antisense drug targeting clusterin, is being evaluated in phase III clinical trials for the treatment of prostate and lung cancers [13]. Also, the antisense drug, AZD9150, which targets signal transducer and activates the transcription 3 (STAT3) in several types of cancers [14] has shown encouraging activity as a single agent in several cancer types. The modified oligonucleotide targeting androgen receptor is in the clinical trial as a possible treatment for prostate cancer [15]. Several additional antisense drugs, including microRNAs and siRNAs, are in early-stage clinical trials.

3.2 Antisense therapy for cardiovascular diseases

The first antisense drug, mipomersen, is approved by the FDA as an adjunct therapy for homozygous familial hypercholesterolemia, which reduces apolipoprotein B mRNA levels [16]. Apolipoprotein C III (apoCIII) plays a critical role in the metabolism of triglyceride-rich lipoproteins, and decreased expression is associated with a lower risk of cardiovascular disease [16, 17]. The clinical trial of volanesorsen, an antisense drug, is designed to reduce apoCIII mRNA levels, and the drug is currently being investigated in placebo-controlled phase III clinical trials for the treatment of familial chylomicronemia syndrome and familial partial lipodystrophy. It has been shown that severe factor XI deficiency provides protection against deep vein thrombosis and therefore cardiovascular morbidity and mortality [6]. The antisense drug IONIS-FXIRx can lower the factor XI levels and has the potential to be more effective than conventional anti-thrombotics. A phase II study with IONIS-FXIRx/BAY 2306001 is ongoing to investigate the drug's effects in patients with end-stage renal disease on hemodialysis [6, 18, 19].

3.3 Antisense therapy for inflammation and autoimmune diseases

The antisense drugs have been and are currently being evaluated for multiple inflammatory diseases, such as inflammatory bowel disease. The oral drug, mongersen targeting the SMAD7 mRNA, showed the promising effects on patients with ulcerative colitis. Also, alicaforsen drug, targeting intercellular adhesion molecule 1 (CD54), has been tested for its effects by systemic delivery in patients with Crohn's disease [20] as well as in the rectal enema patients with ulcerative colitis (or active unremitting pouchitis) [21–23]. This drug is currently being developed for the treatment of chronic refractory pouchitis [21, 24].

3.4 Antisense therapy in neurological disorders

Antisense drugs are being evaluated for multiple neurological diseases and are administered systemically into the cerebrospinal fluid (CSF) that surrounds the brain. Antisense oligonucleotides cannot cross the intact blood–brain barrier efficiently; therefore, they are directly introduced into the CSF or parenchyma to treat brain or spinal cord diseases. Thus, neurological diseases can be approached using different antisense mechanisms and oligonucleotide designs, with single-stranded antisense oligonucleotides and siRNAs used for local therapy [6]. **Duchenne muscular dystrophy** is a progressive, severely disabling, and ultimately lethal neuromuscular disease caused by point mutations, insertions, or chromosomal rearrangements in the dystrophin gene resulting in truncated protein or loss of transcript through nonsense-mediated decay [25]. Because of multiple genomic alterations in Duchenne muscular dystrophy, no single oligonucleotide will address all forms of the disease [6, 25]. Antisense oligonucleotides designed to promote skipping of exon 51 are the most advanced in clinical trials, and the modified phosphorothioate oligonucleotide drug, eteplirsen, is under regulatory review for marketing approval. Additional antisense drugs are currently under development for targeting other exons, which will broaden the treatment of the patient population. **Myotonic dystrophy type 1 (DM1)** is a multisystemic disease caused by a triplet repeat expansion (CTG) in the 3′ untranslated region of myotonic dystrophy protein kinase (DMPK) gene [26]. IONIS-DMPK-2.5Rx is a chimeric antisense oligonucleotide and is currently under a randomized controlled study trail in DM1 patients. **Transthyretin amyloidosis** is a form of systemic amyloidosis caused by misfolded transthyretin protein (TTR), in multiple tissues, including peripheral nerves, the gastrointestinal tract, and the heart [27]. Three different antisense drugs, IONIS-TTRRx, RNase H–dependent, and patisiran, are currently in development for the treatment of TTR amyloidosis, as well as for both familial amyloid polyneuropathy and cardiomyopathy [28]. **Spinal muscular atrophy (SMA)**, a progressive motor neuron disease, usually occurs in infancy or childhood caused by deletions or mutations in the survival of motor neuron 1 (SMN1) gene [29]. Nusinersen drug is a fully modified oligonucleotide designed to bind to a specific sequence in intron 7 of the SMN1 and 2 pre-mRNAs, enhancing exon 7 inclusion and increasing the production of SMN protein [30, 31] which is under review for market authorization. **Huntington's disease (HD)** is an autosomal dominant neurodegenerative disorder resulting from an expanded CAG repeat in the huntingtin (HTT) gene, which causes a toxic gain of function due to an expanded polyglutamine tract in the resulting protein. Antisense oligonucleotide designed to lower total HTT has been shown to provide a prolonged improvement in HD, and the drug is in clinical trial phase [30, 31].

3.5 Antisense therapy for infectious diseases

Various antisense mechanisms can be utilized to inhibit viral replication—for example, by binding to viral mRNA to block the translation of the protein or to degrade the viral RNA through an RNase mechanism or by blocking host microRNAs that support viral replication [6]. Several antisense therapies are currently undergoing clinical trials for various infectious diseases. MicroRNA-122 (miR-122) is highly abundant in the liver and is essential to the stability and propagation of hepatitis C virus (HCV) [32]. This mRNA binds to a highly conserved 5′ untranslated region of the HCV genome, protecting it from degradation and host innate immune responses [32]. Additionally, miR-122 is also believed to play a major role in inflammatory activity in the liver [33], and RG-101, a GalNAc-conjugated oligonucleotide drug, is designed to inhibit miR-122 and HCV replication. The results from this clinical trial were very encouraging and support continued study of the drug.

4. The past, present, and future

The discovery of DNA as hereditary material and the helical structure base paring of DNA have opened the new avenue toward the current understanding and use of nucleic acids for the development of oligonucleotide-based therapies [6, 34]. The antisense oligonucleotides bind to RNA through Watson-Crick base pairing theory and modulate the function of the targeted RNA. This leads to the key discovery and direct importance of development of oligonucleotide-based drugs and medicine [6, 34]. The initial discovery of antisense technology is to enhance or improve the protein and small molecule-based technology by targeting RNA instead of protein. As a therapeutic strategy, it effects the RNA processing and modulates protein expression by binding to RNAs encoding difficult-to-target proteins. However, translating this technology into the clinic had some disadvantage such as inadequate target arrangement, insufficient biological activity, and off-target toxic effects over two decades, but this strategy significantly develops the numbers and types of targets that can be approached for therapy. Further, this technology has a great advantage to develop drugs for the treatment of both monogenic and polygenic diseases as well as influence the human genetics and genomics [12, 34]. The novel chemical modifications of antisense oligonucleotides have been engaged to address these limitations over the years. Both antisense alterations and their mechanism of their action have not only improved the clinical trial design but also provide the breakthrough toward the translation of antisense oligonucleotide-based strategies into therapies [6, 34]. Additionally, multiple clinical trials have clearly confirmed the clinical uses of antisense pharmacology in humans and demonstrated their safety by using various mechanisms. The current antisense drugs, which are under clinical development phase, target different tissues both systemically and locally. The advanced oligonucleotide chemistry further enhances the antisense drug properties by increasing potency, safety, and broader tissue distribution [6]. The advancement of oligonucleotide designs had improved the antisense mechanism of binding to RNA to inhibit their function with and without out RNA degradation. Recently, several researchers demonstrated that antisense oligonucleotides can also be utilized to overexpress or suppress the protein production [34, 35]. Many nonpathogenic disease conditions lack an effective treatment; the rapid development of new improved next-generation antisense oligonucleotide-based drugs bear the potential of intense clinical application and therapeutic impact on the treatment soon, demonstrating that this new class of molecular medicines/drugs has several potential and advantageous applications in the clinic. There was always a lag period from the early discoveries till the therapy enters into the clinical trials and further in the market [34]. RNA-based precision medicine and gene therapy still need the improvement because of their off-target effects. The future applications of antisense technology will solely depend on the performance of novel molecules in the clinical trials. Till date tremendous progress has been made toward the antisense technology, despite the fact this has yet to deliver its full potential [36]. There are still more unanswered questions which need further improvement of the technology. The establishment of first-generation phosphorothioate oligodeoxynucleotides is a great asset and valuable pharmacological tool, which has shown the promise of new therapies to the patient. Further development of new improved second- and third-generation antisense oligonucleotides with novel formulation will result in better therapies for patients. Even though the tremendous progress has been made in antisense technology, there are still more questions that remain unanswered for the technology and opportunities to further improve upon the platform [36]. This technology has provided solutions and confidence to diseases which were earlier considered untreatable. The high-cost factor has prevented this treatment mode inaccessible for the general masses. To fulfill the clinical need, future innovations to this technology might help in finding better and affordable cure to many more diseases which is available to all. Furthermore, the development of CRISPR, an RNA-guided gene-editing technology, and the delivery of mRNA transcribed in vitro are a major development of the RNA therapeutics. The clinical applications and validations of RNA-based antisense drugs for modulation of gene/protein expression and genome editing are currently being investigated both in the laboratory and in the clinic [1]. The CRISPR-Cas genome editing has transformed the field and impacted the biomedical science field which has stimulated the development of RNA-based antisense delivery approaches to facilitate clinical translation of CRISPR-Cas technology [1]. For cancer therapy, the first US-based human trial using CRISPR-Cas9 ex vivo is isolated from the T cells of cancer patients by knocking out the genes encoding PD1 and T-cell receptor alpha/beta [1]. Unquestionably, the field of antisense RNA therapeutics is presently undertaking foremost development, and the potential for using RNA antisense drugs for personalized medicine and immunotherapy as well as to address genetic, infectious, and chronic diseases will ensure the continued development of antisense RNA therapeutics for years to come [1].

5. Summary and conclusion

In summary the antisense oligonucleotides are short, synthetic, single-stranded oligodeoxynucleotides that can alter RNA and reduce, restore, or modify protein expression through several distinct mechanisms by targeting the source of the pathogenesis; antisense-mediated therapies have a higher chance of success than therapies targeting downstream pathways. The advancement in the understanding of antisense pharmacology has provided new energy to translate these therapeutics into the clinic. Further advancement of antisense technology in the clinical settings requires more optimization of antisense delivery, target engagement, and safety profile. This technology holds the potential to change the therapeutic landscape for many disease conditions in near future. Most recently, the first gene therapy-based product, Gendicine (Ad-p53), got approved to treat head and neck squamous cell carcinoma in combination with radiotherapy. Also, the drug, Vitravene (known as fomivirsen), was approved for cytomegalovirus retinitis, Macugen (known as pegaptanib) for age-related macular degeneration, Kynamro (known as mipomersen) for homozygous familial hypercholesterolemia, Exondys 51 (known as eteplirsen) for Duchenne muscular dystrophy, Defitelio (known as defibrotide) for severe hepatic veno-occlusive disease, and Spinraza (known as nusinersen) for spinal muscular atrophy by the FDA. The development of antisense therapeutics has now become a clinical reality. The true advancement in the antisense design, chemistries, synthesis, and delivery technologies has been made for adequate stability, efficacy, specificity, and immune evasion. Finally, antisense technology is beginning to bear fruit.

Author details

Shashwat Sharad[1,2]

1 Center for Prostate Disease Research, Department of Surgery, Uniformed Services University and the Walter Reed National Military Medical Center, Bethesda, Maryland, USA

2 Henry Jackson Foundation for the Advancement of Military Medicine, Bethesda, Maryland, USA

*Address all correspondence to: sharadshashwat@gmail.com

IntechOpen

© 2019 The Author(s). Licensee IntechOpen. This chapter is distributed under the terms of the Creative Commons Attribution License (http://creativecommons.org/licenses/by/3.0), which permits unrestricted use, distribution, and reproduction in any medium, provided the original work is properly cited.

References

[1] Kaczmarek JC, Kowalski PS, Anderson DG. Advances in the delivery of RNA therapeutics: From concept to clinical reality. Genome Medicine. 2017;**9**(1):60

[2] Verdine GL, Walensky LD. The challenge of drugging undruggable targets in cancer: Lessons learned from targeting BCL-2 family members. Clinical Cancer Research. 2007;**13**:7264-7270

[3] Chery J. RNA therapeutics: RNAi and antisense mechanisms and clinical applications. Journal of Postdoctoral Research. 2016;**4**(7):35-50

[4] Ling H. Non-coding RNAs: Therapeutic strategies and delivery systems. Advances in Experimental Medicine and Biology. 2016;**937**:229-237

[5] Bennett CF, Swayze E, Henry S, Geary R. Antisense oligonucleotide-based therapeutics. In: Templeton NS, editor. Gene and Cell Therapy: Therapeutic Mechanisms and Strategies. Boca Raton, FL: CRC Press; 2015. pp. 467-492

[6] Bennett CF, Baker BF, Pham N, Swayze E, Geary RS. Pharmacology of antisense drugs. Annual Review of Pharmacology and Toxicology. 2017;**57**:81-105

[7] Farooqi AA, Rehman ZU, Muntane J. Antisense therapeutics in oncology: Current status. OncoTargets and Therapy. 2014;7:2035-2042

[8] Bennett CF, Swayze EE. RNA targeting therapeutics: Molecular mechanisms of antisense oligonucleotides as a therapeutic platform. Annual Review of Pharmacology and Toxicology. 2010;**50**:259-293

[9] Zhou Y, Zhang C, Liang W. Development of RNAi technology for targeted therapy—A track of siRNA-based agents to RNAi therapeutics. Journal of Controlled Release. 2014;**193**:270-281

[10] Stein CA, Castanotto D. FDA-approved oligonucleotide therapies in 2017. Molecular Therapy. 2017;**25**(5):1069-1075

[11] Piascik P. Fomiversen sodium approved to treat CMV retinitis. Journal of the American Pharmaceutical Association. 1999;**39**:84-85

[12] Krishna M. From petunias to the present- a review of oligonucleotide therapy. Journal of Clinical Epigenetics. 2017;**3**(4):38

[13] Zielinski R, Chi KN. Custirsen (OGX-011): A second-generation antisense inhibitor of clusterin in development for the treatment of prostate cancer. Future Oncology. 2012;**8**:1239-1251

[14] Hong D, Kurzrock R, Kim Y, Woessner R, Younes A, et al. AZD9150, a next-generation antisense oligonucleotide inhibitor of STAT3 with early evidence of clinical activity in lymphoma and lung cancer. Science Translational Medicine. 2015;7:314ra185

[15] Yamamoto Y, Loriot Y, Beraldi E, Zhang F, Wyatt AW, et al. Generation 2.5 antisense oligonucleotides targeting the androgen receptor and its splice variants suppress enzalutamide-resistant prostate cancer cell growth. Clinical Cancer Research. 2015;**21**:1675-1687

[16] Rader DJ, Kastelein JJ. Lomitapide and mipomersen: Two first-in-class drugs for reducing low-density lipoprotein cholesterol in patients with homozygous familial hypercholesterolemia. Circulation. 2014;**129**:1022-1032

[17] Won JI, Zhang J, Tecson KM, McCullough PA. Balancing low-density lipoprotein cholesterol reduction and hepatotoxicity with lomitapide mesylate and mipomersen in patients with homozygous familial hypercholesterolemia. Reviews in Cardiovascular Medicine. 2017;**18**:21-28

[18] Geary RS, Baker BF, Crooke ST. Clinical and preclinical pharmacokinetics and pharmacodynamics of mipomersen (Kynamro): A second-generation antisense oligonucleotide inhibitor of apolipoprotein B. Clinical Pharmacokinetics. 2015;**54**:133-146

[19] Raal FJ, Braamskamp MJ, Selvey SL, Sensinger CH, Kastelein JJP. Pediatric experience with mipomersen as adjunctive therapy for homozygous familial hypercholesterolemia. Journal of Clinical Lipidology. 2016;**10**:860-869

[20] Yacyshyn BR, Chey WY, Wedel MK, Yu RZ, Paul D, Cheung E. A randomized, double-masked, placebo-controlled study of alicaforsen, an antisense inhibitor of intercellular adhesion molecule 1, for the treatment of subjects with active Crohn's disease. Clinical Gastroenterology and Hepatology. 2007;**5**:215-220

[21] Miner P, Wedel M, Bane B, Bradley J. An enema formulation of alicaforsen, an antisense inhibitor of intercellular adhesion molecule-1, in the treatment of chronic, unremitting pouchitis. Alimentary Pharmacology & Therapeutics. 2004;**19**:281-286

[22] Miner PB Jr, Wedel MK, Xia S, Baker BF. Safety and efficacy of two dose formulations of alicaforsen enema compared with mesalazine enema for treatment of mild to moderate left-sided ulcerative colitis: A randomized, double-blind, active-controlled trial. Alimentary Pharmacology & Therapeutics. 2006;**23**:1403-1413

[23] Van Deventer SJH, Wedel MK, Baker BF, Xia S, Chuang E, Miner PB Jr. A phase II dose ranging, double-blind, placebo-controlled study of alicaforsen enema in subjects with acute exacerbation of mild to moderate left-sided ulcerative colitis. Alimentary Pharmacology & Therapeutics. 2006;**23**:1415-1425

[24] Greuter T, Biedermann L, Rogler G, Sauter B, Seibold F. Alicaforsen, an antisense inhibitor of ICAM-1, as treatment for chronic refractory pouchitis after proctocolectomy: A case series. United European Gastroenterology Journal. 2016;**4**:97-104

[25] Flanigan KM. Duchenne and Becker muscular dystrophies. Neurologic Clinics. 2014;**32**:671-688

[26] Brook JD, McCurrach ME, Harley HG, Buckler AJ, Church D, et al. Molecular basis of myotnic dystrophy: Expansion of a trinucleotides (CTG) repeat at the 3 -end of a transcript encoding a protein kinase family member. Cell. 1992;**68**:799-808

[27] Gertz MA, Benson MD, Dyck PJ, Grogan M, Coelho T, et al. Diagnosis, prognosis, and therapy of transthyretin amyloidosis. Journal of the American College of Cardiology. 2015;**66**:2451-2466

[28] Ackermann EJ, Guo S, Benson MD, Booten S, Freier S, et al. Suppressing transthyretin production in mice, monkeys and humans using 2nd-generation antisense oligonucleotides. Amyloid. 2016;**23**:148-157

[29] Lefebvre S, Burlet P, Liu Q, Bertrandy S, Clermont O, et al. Correlation between severity and SMN protein level in spinal muscular atrophy. Nature Genetics. 1997;**16**:265-269

[30] Passini MA, Bu J, Richards AM, Kinnecom C, Sardi SP, et al. Antisense oligonucleotides delivered to the mouse CNS ameliorate symptoms of severe spinal muscular atrophy. Science Translational Medicine. 2011;**3**:72ra18

[31] Hua Y, Sahashi K, Hung G, Rigo F, Passini MA, et al. Antisense correction of SMN2 splicing in the CNS rescues necrosis in a type III SMA mouse model. Genes & Development. 2010;**24**:1634-1644

[32] Jopling CL, Yi M, Lancaster AM, Lemon SM, Sarnow P. Modulation of hepatitis C virus RNA abundance by a liver-specific microRNA. Science. 2005;**309**:1577-1581

[33] van der Meer AJ, Farid WR, Sonneveld MJ, de Ruiter PE, Boonstra A, et al. Sensitive detection of hepatocellular injury in chronic hepatitis C patients with circulating hepatocyte-derived microRNA-122. Journal of Viral Hepatitis. 2013;**20**:158-166

[34] Lundin KE, Gissberg O, Smith CI. Oligonucleotide therapies: The past and the present. Human Gene Therapy. 2015;**26**(8):475-485

[35] Geary RS, Norris D, Yu R, et al. Pharmacokinetics, bio distribution and cell uptake of antisense oligonucleotides. Advanced Drug Delivery Reviews. 2015;**87**:46-51

[36] Gulam M, Khan NJ, Maheshwari KK, Porwal M. Antisense therapy and its application in biopharmaceutical research: Past, present and future. Asian Pacific Journal of Applied Sciences. 2016:61-69. ISSN: 2456-1622

Chapter 2

Antisense Oligonucleotides, A Novel Developing Targeting Therapy

Sara Karaki, Clément Paris and Palma Rocchi

Abstract

Antisense oligonucleotides (ASOs) have been validated as therapeutic agents and an important tool in molecular biology. Indeed, ASOs are used either *in vitro* or *in vivo* to generate mRNA selective knockouts. They can be used for human therapy since ASOs can inhibit specifically target genes especially whose are difficult to target with small molecules inhibitors or neutralizing antibodies. However, despite their specificity and broadness of use, some practical obstacles remain unsolved in antisense pharmacology, such as insufficient stability due to nucleases degradation activity, and poor cellular delivery as a result of low cellular uptake difficult biological membrane crossing. Moreover, in many cases, potential off-target effects and immunostimulation are also part of the problems derived from their use. In this review, we will discuss ASOs, their chemistry, limitation of use, some solutions to increase stability, and finally some of their therapeutical application.

Keywords: antisense oligonucleotide, ASO chemistry, ASO delivery, therapeutic target, cancer

1. Introduction

The usage of nucleic acids in therapeutics is founded on the inhibition of RNA expression and on their capacity to modulate the expression of a target protein associate to a disease [1]. ASOs are typically modified synthetic nucleic acids. They are single stand oligonucleotide with 16-mer to 21-mer sequence with high affinity for a specific RNA target sequence, through base pairing [2]. The two general chemical classes of nucleic acids commonly used today are antisense oligonucleotides (ASOs) and siRNA. The first is single-stranded, and modulates RNA function either by degrading the RNA sequence in question due to enzyme RNase H activity, or by modifying splicing function thus affecting RNA metabolism; and the second is double-stranded synthetic oligonucleotides that degrade target RNA through an RNA-induced silencing complex (RISC). Importantly, both must reach the nucleus and/or cytoplasm to exert their activity, and thus must cross a biological membrane.

Although ASOs and siRNA share similarities, they are divergent on some points, and so, choosing ASO or siRNA strategy for gene targeting depends on the target gene. However, since ASOs are single stranded, as opposed to siRNA, they have lower cost of production. Moreover, it is easier to deliver ASOs *in vivo*, since they do not a vector and a simple chemical modification can increase their resistance to nucleases, as opposed to siRNA that need a carrier. Finally, for *in vitro* studies, siRNA is considered a better technology, since it's relatively easier to obtain a potent siRNA since unmodified RNA works with high potency as opposed to ASOs.

In this review we will mainly focus on ASOs chemistry and mechanism of action.

Indeed, since Zamecnik in 1978 used an ASO-like unmodified DNA sequence in cell culture, notable progress has been made in ASO pharmacology [3]. Currently, the efficacy of different ASOs is being studied in many neurodegenerative diseases such as Huntington's disease, Parkinson's disease, Alzheimer's disease, and amyotrophic lateral sclerosis but also in several cancer states. Numerous ASO-based therapeutics are being tested in clinical trials. In **Table 1** figures some of the ASO in clinical trial for cancer treatments. However, until now, only two ASOs have been approved by the US FDA to be used on humans, namely, fomivirsen (Vitravene),

Study id; year; country of conduct of study	Sponsors	Disease conditions	Phase of clinical trial; target mRNA
NCT00063934; 2003; USA	National Cancer Institute (NCI)	Breast cancer	Phase 1/2; Bcl-2
NCT01563302; 2012; USA	Isis Pharmaceuticals	Lymphoma	Phase 1/2; STAT 3
NCT01839604; 2013; Hong Kong	AstraZeneca	Metastatic hepatocellular carcinoma	Phase 1; STAT-3
NCT00258375; 2005; USA	NCIC Clinical Trials Group	Metastatic breast cancer	cancer Phase 2; Clusterin
NCT00070083; 2003; United Kingdom	British Columbia Cancer Agency	Diffuse large B cell lymphoma	Phase 1; Bcl-2
NCT02549651; 2015; USA	MedImmune LLC	Diffuse large B-cell lymphoma	Phase 1; STAT 3 NCT02243124; 2014;
NCT00030641; 2002; USA	Genta Incorporated	Non small cell lung cancer	Phase 2/3; Bcl-2
NCT00070343; 2003; USA	Jonsson Comprehensive Cancer Center	Malignant melanoma	Bcl-2
NCT01780545; 2013; USA	OncoGenex Technologies	Metastatic bladder cancer	Phase 2; Heat shock protein 27
NCT00085228; 2004; Belgium	European Organisation for Research and Treatment of Cancer	Adenocarcinoma prostate	Phase 2; Bcl-2
NCT00543205; 2007; USA	Genta Incorporated	Melanoma	Melanoma Phase 2/3; Bcl-2
NCT00054106; 2003; USA	NCIC Clinical Trials Group	Prostate cancer	Phase 1; Bcl-2
NCT01120470; 2010; United Kingdom	British Columbia Cancer Agency	Castration resistant prostate cancer	Phase 2; Heat shock protein-27
NCT00636545; 2007; USA	Genta Incorporated	Solid tumours	Phase 1; Bcl-2
NCT00896857; 2009; USA	Cancer Center of Wake Forest University	Breast cancer	Bcl-2
NCT01083615; 2010; USA	OncoGenex Technologies	Prostate cancer	Phase 3; Clusterin
NCT02144051; 2014; USA	AstraZeneca	Advanced solid tumours with androgen receptor pathway as a potential factor	Phase 1; Androgen receptor

Table 1.
Registered clinical studies with ASO in cancer treatments in clinical trials.gov.

a first-generation ASO for cytomegalovirus (CMV) retinitis, and mipomersen (Kynamro), a second-generation ASO for homozygous familial hypercholesterolemia (HoFH) [4, 5], both developed by Isis Pharmaceuticals. They work via RNase H-mediated cleavage of the targeted RNA.

2. ASO's design, chemistry and mechanism of action

2.1 ASO's mechanism of action

Two major mechanisms contribute to the antisense activity. The first is that most ASOs are designed to activate RNase H, which cleaves the RNA moiety of a DNA–RNA heteroduplex and therefore leads to degradation of the target mRNA in the nucleus and cytoplasm. In addition, ASOs that do not induce RNase H cleavage can be used to inhibit translation by steric blockade of the ribosome in the cytoplasm [6]. When the ASOs are targeted to the 5′-terminus, binding and assembly of the translation machinery can be prevented [7]. Most mammalian RNAs undergo multiple post-transcriptional processing steps in the cell nucleus including addition of a 5′-cap structure, splicing and polyadenylation.

Regulation of RNA processing is another efficient mechanism in which ASOs can be utilized to regulate gene expression. Studies have been published documenting that ASOs can be used to destabilize pre-mRNA [8] and to regulate RNA splicing [9]. Another viable approach to reversibly 'switch' protein function is alternative splicing that generates RNA encoding antagonistic proteins (**Figure 1**). Whether RNaseH activity takes place favorably in the cytoplasm or in the nucleus is not well documented. However, most studies suggest that the most part of the inhibition takes place in the cytoplasm. Controversially, ASOs that targets pre-mRNA and are splice modulators are active in the nucleus.

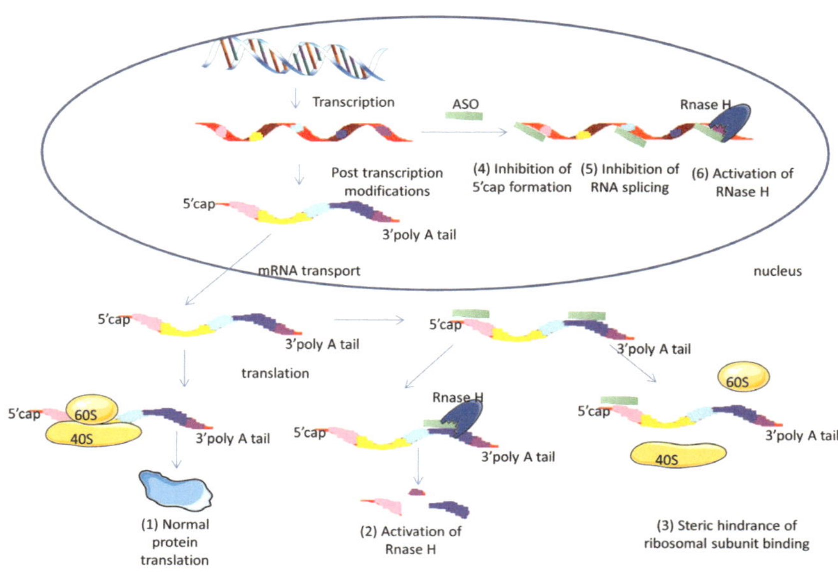

Figure 1.
ASOs mechanism of action. (1) In the absence of ASO, normal gene and protein expression is maintained. (2) Formation of ASO-mRNA heteroduplex in cytoplasm induces activation of RNase H, leading to mRNA degradation or (3) steric interference of ribosomal assembly. Alternatively, ASO can enter the nucleus and regulate mRNA maturation by (4) inhibition of 5′ cap formation, (5) inhibition of mRNA splicing and (6) activation of RNase H.

2.2 ASO's design

There are several screening strategies to obtain potent ASO, such as using a computational algorithm in ASO design [10], mRNA walking [11], OD array [12] and RNase H mapping [13]. However, some of these approaches are labor intensive and require expensive automation equipment. Many factors can affect the strength and stability of the ASO-mRNA interaction, such as the mRNA secondary structure, thermodynamic stability and also the position of the hybridization site relative to functional motifs on the target RNA, such as the 5' CAP region or translational start site.

To find a highly potent ASO, the "hit rate" can be increased by considering four parameters during ASO design:

2.2.1 Prediction of the secondary structure of the RNA

It is recognized that a secondary structure of the RNA accurately predicted, leads to effective ASO design [14, 15]. Some algorithm able to predict any single mRNA secondary structure and folding pattern are currently available, such as the *m*fold and the *s*fold program.

2.2.2 Identification of preferable RNA secondary local structures

In order for the ASO to be effective, it should target mRNA regions accessible to hybridization [16], such as joint sequences, internal loops, and hairpins of 10 or more consecutive nucleotides, usually located at the terminal end of the sequence [17]. It has been shown that highly conserved motifs are a good target of a potent ASO, whereas ASO targeting variable local motifs may induce non-sequence specific effects [18]. Therefore, the best approach to increase the 'hit rate' of potent ASO design is to target these conserved motifs among several optimal mRNA predicted secondary structures.

2.2.3 Motifs searching and GC content calculation

Although RNase activity is stimulated by the formation of the ASO-mRNA heteroduplex, leading to the mRNA degradation, it has been shown that this activity occurs independently of the ASO sequence, but is rather strongly correlated to the GC content which is also known to affect thermodynamic stability.

The perfect content of GC is still controversial; it is described that a strong ASO effect is observed with a percentage of 45–65% of G or C residues [10]; however, many of the ASOs used in therapy today do not have a GC content in this range.

2.2.4 Binding energy prediction

Thermodynamic energy is also important to a successful ASO design. Some available software can calculate thermodynamic properties between the target mRNA sequence and the ASO. To design a potent ASO, the binding energy between the ASO and mRNA should be $DG37 \geq -8$ kcal/mol, whereas the energy for binding between ASOs should be $DG37 \geq -1.1$ kcal/mol [19].

2.3 ASO's chemical modification

The use of unmodified ASOs is limited as they have an overall charged property that prevents them from getting through the cell membrane and are rapidly attacked by all types of intracellular endonucleases and exonucleases, usually via 3′-5′ activity in biological fluid. In addition, the degradation products of phosphodiester ODs may be cytotoxic and also exert anti-proliferative effects. Moreover, some unspecific hybridization has been observed and finally for most applications immunostimulation has also been a matter of concern [20, 21]. This part will be further detailed in the toxicity chapter.

Numerous chemical modifications have been developed to improve nuclease resistance, extend tissue half-life, reduce non-sequence-specific toxicity, as well as to increase affinity and potency (**Figure 2**).

2.3.1 First-generation ASO

First-generation ASOs are the ones having a phosphorothioate (PTO) modified backbone. These ASOs have a sulfur atom that substitutes the non-bridging oxygen atoms in the phosphodiester bond [22] (**Figure 2a**). PTO modification confers higher resistance to the ASO against nuclease degradation, leading to higher bioavailability. Additionally, they are highly soluble and have excellent antisense activity [23]. Finally, PTO-modified ASOs promote degradation of target mRNA by RNase H enzyme. Nevertheless, this modification may slightly reduce the affinity of the ASO for its mRNA target because the melting temperature (Tm) of the ASO-mRNA heteroduplex is decreased [20]. PTO modification is the most widely

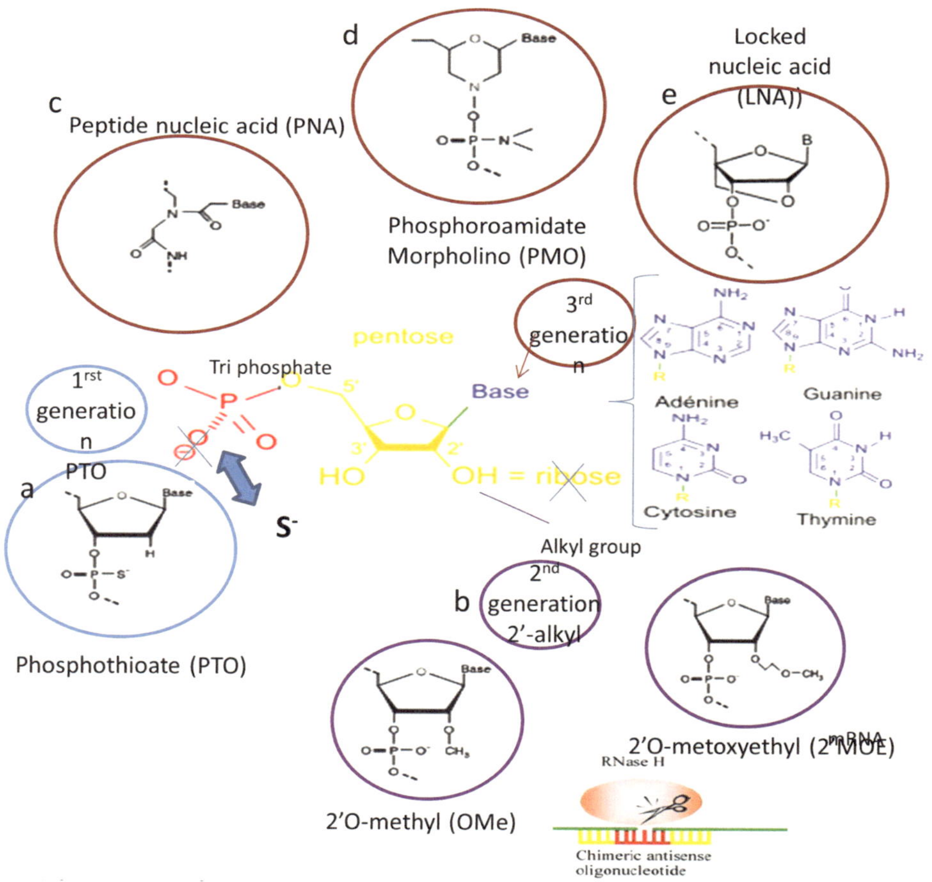

Figure 2.
Chemical modifications of ASO. (a) First-generation PTO, (b) second generation, RNase H cleavage induced by chimeric ASO, and (c–e) third-generation ASO.

performed chemical modification of ASOs for loss-of-function studies *in vitro* and *in vivo* for gene target identification and validation. These data have led to the introduction of PTO ASOs into clinical therapeutic trials. Indeed, Fomivirsen, a currently FDA approved drug for clinical use, is a first-generation PTO-modified ASO [24]. Despite the fact the PTO modifications are the most widely used ODs, they have many properties which render them suboptimal antisense effector molecules. The PTO backbone is known to induce sequence-independent effects attributable to its length dependent high affinity for various cellular proteins. However, this seemingly negative property of PTO ASOs to interact with certain proteins proved to be advantageous for the pharmacokinetic profile. Their binding to plasma proteins protects them from filtration and is responsible for an increased serum half-life [25]. Finally, these oligonucleotides can interact with components of the innate immune system such as Toll-like receptors (TLRs), inducing an immune response and triggering cytokines expression and other genes coding for the nonspecific defense mechanisms [26].

Nevertheless, to try to solve the several non-specific problems [27], new chemical modifications have been developed. Modifications to the base, sugar and backbone have been identified that increase binding affinity for the target RNA.

2.3.2 Second-generation ASO

The second generation represents oligonucleotides in which the structural modification is not limited to the backbone linkage but additionally includes structural modifications of the ribose: ASO with 2'-O-alkyl modifications of the ribose were developed (**Figure 2b**). These modifications intend to improve binding affinity, to increase efficacy, to modulate the protein binding of oligonucleotides and to enhance nuclease resistance. 2'-O-Methyl (2'-OMe) and 2'-O-Methoxyethyl (2'-MOE) modifications of ASO-PTO are the most widely studied [28]. These second-generation ASOs are less toxic than PTO- modified ASOs and have a slightly enhanced affinity towards their complementary RNAs [29]. Moreover, an important aspect for these ASOs is that 2'modifications can reduce immunostimulatory effect [30]. However, 2'-OMe and 2'-MOE substitutions do not activate the RNase H to cleave the target mRNA, which decreases the efficacy of the ASO [31]. Indeed, mechanistic studies have been conducted to elucidate RNase H activity. They have shown that the flexibility of the ASO, the accessibility of the 2′-OH group of the RNA and the correct width of the minor groove of the ASO-RNA duplex are necessary for effective RNase H mediated mRNA degradation [32]. Since 2′-*O*-alkyl RNA ODs do not activate the RNase H, they inhibit mRNA expression only by a steric interference with translation. However, to increase its potency, an ASO should be able to induce cleavage by RNase H. Therefore, a chimeric ASO was developed (**Figure 2b**). It consists of a central 'gap' region containing 10 DNA or PTO DNA monomers and flanked on both sides (5'and 3'extremities) by approximatively 5 modified nucleotides such as 2′-OM or 2'-MOE (indicated by red and yellow regions of the OD in **Figure 2b**). This chimeric 'gapmer' ASO allows RNase H to sit in the central gap and to execute target-specific mRNA degradation; meanwhile, the flanking 2′-alkyl modified ends prevent nuclease cleavage of ASO. The 2′-*O*-MOE-PTO gapmers OGX-427 (Apatorsen) developed by Rocchi et al., directed against HSP27 and OGX-011 (Curtisen) against clusterin are currently undergoing clinical trials (**Table 1**). The ODs being tested clinically mainly incorporate relatively simple chemical modifications such as the PTO modifications and the 2′-alkyl modifications (first- and second-generation ODs).

DOI: http://dx.doi.org/10.5772/intechopen.82105

2.3.3 Third-generation ASO

Third-generation ASOs have been developed to further improve nuclease resistance, increase binding affinity, and to enhance pharmacokinetics and biostability. They are characterized by chemical modifications of the nucleotide, and more precisely to its furanose ring [33]. Many modifications have been described, such as N3′-P5′ phosphoramidates, 2′-deoxy-2′-fluoro-β-D-arabino nucleic acid analogue (FANA), cyclohexene nucleic acids (CeNAs) and tricyclo-DNA (tcDNA), however, peptide nucleic acid (PNA), phosphoramidate morpholino oligomer (PMO) and locked nucleic acid (LNA) are the three most studied third-generation ASOs [34, 35].

It should be noted that there is no single modification that covers all the desired properties for a modified ASO. As described before, chemical modifications can improve ASO-RNA hybridization affinity, enhance nuclease resistance, decrease toxicity and modulate pharmacokinetics. An optimal antisense can be designed depending on its use by mixing and matching the numerous chemical modifications accordingly.

2.3.3.1 Peptide nucleic acid

PNA is a synthetic DNA mimic in which the deoxyribose phosphate backbone is replaced by polyamide linkages [36] (**Figure 2c**). PNAs are biologically very stable and have good hybridization properties. However, they do not activate mRNA cleavage via RNase activity, but rather block translation and thus protein expression, by forming sequence-specific duplex with mRNA, hence generating steric hindrance. Due to their neutral backbone, PNAs have low solubility and their cellular uptake remains a challenge for exploiting them as therapeutics antisense. PNAs delivery can be enhanced annealing a PNA strand with a negatively charged complementary oligonucleotide, and then enclosed the obtained duplex with a cationic lipid. To this end, PNAs are also conjugated to peptides for improving their cellular uptake [37, 38]. Furthermore, PNA can elicit antigen effects by hybridizing with double-stranded DNA [36, 39] resulting in transcriptional arrest. Substantial data have revealed the effectiveness of PNA in gene silencing in various in vitro models [39, 40].

2.3.3.2 Phosphoramidate morpholino oligomer

PMOs are non-charged ASOs whose pentose sugar is substituted by a morpholino ring and the inter-nucleotide linkages are phosphoramidate bonds in place of phosphodiester bonds [41] (**Figure 2d**). PMOs avoid the RNase H recruitment; their effect is primarily mediated by steric interference of ribosomal assembly resulting in translational arrest. Synthetic PMOs are resistant to nucleases degradation in biological fluid. Because their backbone is uncharged, PMOs are unlikely to form unwanted interactions with nucleic acid-binding proteins [42]. PMOs do not enter mammalian cells easily in culture, but it has been shown that conjugating it with peptides such as arginine-rich peptide (ARP) can enhance its cellular uptake and antisense potency [43]. Antisense PMO oligonucleotide, have shown efficacy in animal models *in vivo* and in human clinical trials [44, 45]. Indeed, a PMO antisense agent is currently in phase II clinical trials for restenosis, cancer and polycystic kidney disease.

2.3.3.3 Locked nucleic acid

Locked nucleic acids oligonucleotides figure among the most promising candidates developed the last few years. LNAs are chemically modified nucleotides with a ribose containing a methylene bridge between the 2′-oxygen and the 4′-carbon

	Nuclease stability	Cellular uptake	Charge	RNase activity
PTO	+	+/-	negative	++
2'OME, 2'MOE	+	+/-	negative	Chimeric: +
PNA	+	-	0	- Steric hindrance
PMO	+	-	0	- steric interference with ribosomes
LNA	+	-	0	Chimeric +

Table 2.
Chemical modification characteristics.

of the ribose [46]. LNA modifications improve significantly the ASO hybridization affinity towards mRNA target, due to the important increase in the thermal stability of the DNA/RNA heteroduplexes [47]. In addition, LNAs avoid nuclease degradation. As their ribose 2'-O position are modified, LNAs are not recruiting RNase H [48]. Nevertheless LNA nucleotides can be freely incorporated at the ends of RNA and DNA sequences to form chimeric oligonucleotides resulting in restoration of RNase H-mediated cleavage of mRNA. It has been shown that the chimeric LNA/DNA/LNA gapmer with seven to 10 phosphorothioate-modified DNA central gaps flanked by three to four LNA nucleotides on both 5′-end and 3'ends induces efficient mRNA cleavage, because of their high target affinity and nuclease resistance [29]. In the first *in vivo* study reported, the LNA ASOs appeared to be nontoxic in the optimal dosage. Therefore, full LNA and gapmers LNA·DNA·LNA ASOs seem to offer an attractive set of properties, such as potent biological activity and apparent lack of acute toxicity, making it a promising antisense agents [49–51]. **Table 2** recapitulates the chemical modifications characteristics.

Despite the large number of molecules being evaluated in the clinical trials, the clinical progress of ASOs had to face many challenges; indeed, poor pharmacokinetics [52], poor cell membrane permeation [53], and off-target effects [27]. Last decade, the development of oligonucleotide delivery through lipid or polymer systems has improved the cellular uptake and the pharmacokinetic behavior [54].

3. ASO's pharmacokinetics, toxicity and delivery

3.1 ASO's pharmacokinetics and toxicity

The pharmacokinetics of ASOs has been extensively studied; they rapidly distribute to all tissues *in vivo* [55]. First and second-generation PTO ODs are broadly distributed to all peripheral tissues. The highest concentrations of ODs are found in the liver, kidney, spleen, lymph nodes and bone marrow with no measurable distribution to the brain [52]. Moreover, they not only distribute to tissues but also accumulate within cells in tissues [56]. The mechanism(s) by which ODs accumulate within cells following parenteral administration is currently unknown [57]. However, ODs that do not contain a PTO linkage appear to be rapidly excreted in the urine [58]. This difference in tissue distribution appears to be due largely to interactions with plasma proteins.

In summary, pharmacokinetic studies of PTO ASO demonstrate that they are well absorbed from parenteral sites, distribute broadly to all peripheral tissues, do not cross the blood-brain barrier (BBB), and are eliminated primarily by slow metabolism. Altogether, their pharmacokinetic properties depend on chemistry rather than sequence.

Concerning ASO's toxicity, there are two broad categories of potential toxicities for ASOs; toxicities due to exaggerated pharmacology and toxicities due to non-antisense effects of the ASO. The former category of side effects results from the ASO binding to off-target RNA, producing an undesirable effect. The potential for such toxicities can be further minimized by vigilant selection of the drug target and homology searches against human genomic databases. The second category of potential toxicities (non-antisense effects) has been documented at higher doses of ASOs. In clinical trials PTO ASOs have proven to be safer than originally anticipated [31, 34, 35]. ASOs drugs principally induce mild-to-moderate toxicities related to the administered dose. *In vivo,* the two mains mechanism that induce acute toxicity through ASOs administration are for the first one the activation of the transient complement cascade and for the second one the inhibition of the clotting cascade. The increase in the clotting times is defined by a transient concentration-dependent escalation of activated partial thromboplastin times (aPTT) [59]. Another frequently occurring sub chronic toxicity is immune stimulation, manifested as splenomegaly, lymphoid hyperplasia and diffused multi-organ mixed mononuclear cell infiltrates [60]. This is due to an unmethylated cytosine-phosphorous-guanine (CpG) motif in the ASO sequence that can be recognized by Toll-like receptor (TLR)-9 in immune cells. This results in the release of cytokines, interleukin (IL)-6, IL-12, interferon (INF)-γ), B cell proliferation, antibody production and activation of T lymphocyte and natural killer (NK) cells [61]. In order to avoid the immune response, the cytosine of the sequences including CpG motif are substituted by methylated cytosine. Also, for preventing this side-effect, the sequences of ASOs drug can be designed without CpG motif. These both stimulatory immune responses are related to the sequence and the chemical modification of the ASOs [6]. Indeed, second-generation ASOs have been shown to have smaller immune stimulation that ASOs PTO. In addition, introduction of LNA into the PTO-ASO has been shown to reduce, and even eliminate, CpG dinucleotide-mediated immunostimulation [62, 63]. When ASO's plasma concentration is high, some toxicities have been observed, such as elevated liver enzyme such as aspartate aminotransferase (AST) and alanine amino-transferase (ALT), thrombocytopenia, and hyperglycemia [52].

3.2 ASO's delivery

Although the clinical relevance of ASOs has been demonstrated, inefficient cellular uptake, both *in vitro* and *in vivo*, limit the efficacy of ASOs and has been a barrier to therapeutic development. Cellular uptake can be <2% of the dose resulting in too low ASO concentration at the active site for an effective and sustained outcome [22]. Indeed, many researches are conducted on the improvement of ASO delivery via the use of delivery vehicles.

3.2.1 Mechanism of cellular uptake

Cellular uptake refers to the combination of both OD membrane-binding and internalization. It is challenged by numerous barriers, most importantly, the lipophilic nature of the cell membrane, which makes the passage of these large anionic molecules complicated. Several barriers to cellular uptake exist such as the lipophilic cell membrane, through which these large, anionic molecules must pass to reach the site of action. In cultured cells, the internalization of naked ASOs is generally inefficient, with only a few ASO molecules actually penetrating the cell [21]. Exogenously administered ASOs enter cells *in vitro* by a combination of fluid-phase (pinocytosis), caveolae potocytosis, adsorptive and receptor-mediated endocytosis (**Figure 3**), cellular uptake mechanisms being different depending on the ASO chemical structure. However, this results in a trafficking problem because not all of the internalized ASO will be able to reach their target and interact with it. This is because the majority of internalized ASO is sequestered into endosome or lysosomal compartments [21]. A significant amount of the OD is also compartmentalized within other cellular organelles, such as the Golgi complex and the endoplasmic reticulum [64].

To improve cellular uptake and OD's activity, a range of techniques and transporters have been developed [65, 66]. Simultaneously, the use of these vectors increases the stability of ODs against nuclease digestion and allows the use of lower concentrations of ODs.

3.2.2 General delivery methods

OD delivery can occur through carrier molecules. Receptor-mediated endocytosis-directed uptake utilizes import mechanisms already present in the cell membrane for the uptake of biomolecules necessary for cell function [67]. ODs can be linked directly to a carrier protein *via* a covalent bond or non-covalently via poly-L-lysine (PLL)-carrier conjugates. The choice of the carrier is dependent on its known ability to bind to specific cell membrane receptors and accumulate in the cell via endocytosis. Not only OD's internalization can be potentially improved, but cell-specific delivery can also be achieved by targeting receptors exclusively expressed or over-expressed on certain target cells. However, the OD is generally sequestrated in endosomal compartments, thereby limiting the utility of this method for delivery [22]. The use of peptides can help overcome this issue. Indeed, as peptides have membrane translocation properties, they can increase ODs passage through the plasma membrane. For example, fusogenic peptides have been used to promote peptide fusion of OD-peptide conjugates with either cell or lysosomal membranes [68]. To facilitate OD transport to the nucleus, nuclear localization signals (NLS) can be used for ODs that inhibit pre mRNA splicing [69]. Another peptide used is CPP, a short peptide sequence

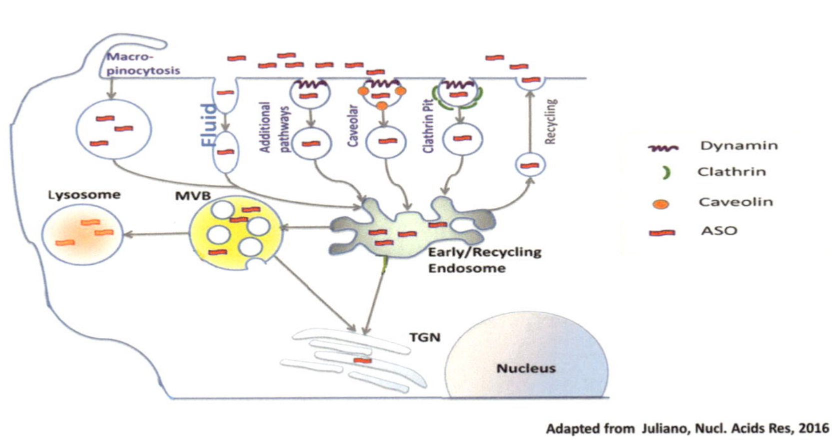

Figure 3.
Cellular uptake and intracellular trafficking of oligonucleotides. Oligonucleotides enter cells via several endocytotic pathways. Most of ODs are recycled in early recycling endosomes. ODs accumulate in endosomes, multivesicular bodies (MVB) and lysosomes. A significant amount is compartmentalized in cellular organelles like the trans Golgi network (TGN).

(<30 amino acids) with net positive charge that uses an energy dependent pathway to allow internalization of large molecules like ASOs. Commonly used CPP include penetratin, HIV TAT peptide and transportan. Through disulfide bond, ASOs and CPP can be conjugated. To evaluate ASO-CPP effect on mRNA degradation *in vitro* and *in vivo,* PNA is the most used [43, 70, 71]. An interesting variation is to couple two different ASOs to a single CPP thus addressing two targets simultaneously [72]. The most dramatic advance in OD targeting has involved delivery *via* the asialoglycoprotein receptors (ASGR). ASGPR, also known as the Ashwell receptor, is a lectin that is abundantly expressed on hepatocytes [73] and clears serum glycoproteins by receptor-mediated endocytosis [74]. The functional receptor is a trimer comprised of two proteins and exhibits high affinity for *N*-acetyl galactosamine (GalNAc) terminated oligosaccharides [75]. A major breakthrough came from researchers who developed multivalent GalNac conjugated siRNAs that bind to the ASGR [76]. The conjugates were effectively taken up into primary mouse hepatocytes by a receptor-specific mechanism, leading to silencing of targeted genes. GalNac based conjugates have similarly been used to transport ASOs to the liver in mice with good effects on reduction of target gene expression [77]. Indeed, GalNac-ASOs showed high affinity for mouse ASGPR, which resulted in enhanced ASO delivery to hepatocytes. Furthermore, once inside the cell, GalNac-ASO's metabolism leads to ASO release in the liver, thus acting like a prodrug targeting hepatocytes. Moreover it improved potency and extent the effect of both antisense targeting human transthyretin (TTR) and human apolipoprotein C-III in transgenic mice. This study highlighted several of the virtues of conjugates including use of a molecularly defined entity, high tissue and cell selectivity and lack of substantial toxicity. The successes with glycoconjugates in the laboratory have facilitated their rapid translation to clinical evaluation, with several hepatic genes being addressed. Finally, an additional approach to OD internalization is to generate transient permeabilization of the plasma membrane and allow naked ODs to penetrate into the cells by diffusion. It consists of inducing transitory pores in the membrane, either chemically by streptolysin-O-permeabilization, mechanically by microinjection, or by electroporation [78] or ultrasound.

All of these methods, under defined circumstances, can permit charged or uncharged ODs to enter cells rapidly and localize in the nucleus, where they produce antisense inhibition of gene function.

Nevertheless, one of the most promising strategies used to overcome cellular barriers is the use of nanotechnology. Indeed, nanocarriers offer the possibility to encapsulate drugs but also nucleic acid, to protect it from degradation, enhance its distribution to the tissues and the cells, but also reduce toxicity and thus secondary effects by targeting specific organs. It is a very promising tool for combination therapy and theranostics applications. To bypass the limitations of ASO-based therapy, like insufficient stability and low intracellular delivery and distribution, Dr. Rocchi's lab recently developed a modified first-generation ASO by using a lipid-conjugated oligonucleotide modification (LASO) able to overcome the problems to ASO administration. The idea is to improve ASO's stability, efficiency and biodisponibility by adding a hydrophobic lipid chain at the 5'end of the hydrophilic DNA sequence. As amphiphiles, LASOs self-assemble in aqueous media with an encapsulation rate of 100%, which yields in small spherical objects of ~11 nm in diameter [79]. Due to their small size, these nanomicelles, can accumulate inside the tumor *via* EPR effect (enhanced permeability and retention effect), which permits passive targeting and reduced systemic toxicity. Interestingly, transfection with these lipid-modified ASO leads to rapid and prolonged internalization *via* micropinocytosis with no transfecting agent. Interestingly, the addition of the lipid, does not affect LASO's efficacy *in vitro* and *in vivo* with little or no toxicity in animal models.

4. Discussion/conclusion

Antisense oligonucleotide based therapies are promising. They can be used for human therapy and can specifically inhibit target genes. Despite the promising progress since their discovery, only a few have been approved for clinical use. This low success rate can be explained by their anionic charge which prevents them from getting through the cell membrane and are rapidly destroyed by nuclease. To address these problems many chemical modifications have been developed. Finally, improvement of their delivery to the tissues, and thus their efficacy is an important issue that has to be addressed. To solve this problem, many strategies have been studied; nanotechnology is one of the most promising to overcome the cellular barriers for the ASO delivery towards targeted therapy.

Author details

Sara Karaki, Clément Paris and Palma Rocchi*
CRCM: Aix Marseille Université, CNRS, INSERM, Institut Paoli-Calmettes, CRCM, Marseille, France

*Address all correspondence to: palma.rocchi@inserm.fr

IntechOpen

© 2019 The Author(s). Licensee IntechOpen. This chapter is distributed under the terms of the Creative Commons Attribution License (http://creativecommons.org/licenses/by/3.0), which permits unrestricted use, distribution, and reproduction in any medium, provided the original work is properly cited.

References

[1] Sridharan K, Gogtay NJ. Therapeutic nucleic acids: Current clinical status. British Journal of Clinical Pharmacology. 2016 Sep;**82**(3):659-672

[2] Cavagnari BM. Gene therapy: Nucleic acids as drugs. Action mechanisms and delivery into the cell. Archivos Argentinos de Pediatría. 2011 Jun; **109**(3):237-244

[3] Zamecnik PC, Stephenson ML. Inhibition of Rous sarcoma virus replication and cell transformation by a specific oligodeoxynucleotide. Proceedings of the National Academy of Sciences of the United States of America. 1978 Jan;**75**(1):280-284

[4] Grillone LR, Lanz R. Fomivirsen. Drugs Today (Barc). 2001 Apr;**37**(4):245-255

[5] Wong E, Goldberg T. Mipomersen (kynamro): A novel antisense oligonucleotide inhibitor for the management of homozygous familial hypercholesterolemia. Pharmacy and Therapeutics. 2014 Feb;**39**(2):119-122

[6] Bennett CF, Swayze EE. RNA targeting therapeutics: Molecular mechanisms of antisense oligonucleotides as a therapeutic platform. Annual Review of Pharmacology and Toxicology. 2010;**50**:259-293

[7] Wu H, Lima WF, Zhang H, Fan A, Sun H, Crooke ST. Determination of the role of the human RNase H1 in the pharmacology of DNA-like antisense drugs. The Journal of Biological Chemistry. 2004 Apr;**279**(17):17181-17189

[8] Kole R, Krainer AR, Altman S. RNA therapeutics: Beyond RNA interference and antisense oligonucleotides. Nature Reviews. Drug Discovery. 2012 Feb;**11**(2):125-140

[9] Disterer P, Kryczka A, Liu Y, Badi YE, Wong JJ, Owen JS, et al. Development of therapeutic splice-switching oligonucleotides. Human Gene Therapy. 2014 Jul;**25**(7):587-598

[10] Chan JH, Lim S, Wong WS. Antisense oligonucleotides: From design to therapeutic application. Clinical and Experimental Pharmacology & Physiology. 2006 May-Jun;**33**(5-6):533-540

[11] Sohail M, Southern EM. Selecting optimal antisense reagents. Advanced Drug Delivery Reviews. 2000 Oct;**44**(1):23-34

[12] Cho YS, Kim MK, Cheadle C, Neary C, Becker KG, Cho-Chung YS. Antisense DNAs as multisite genomic modulators identified by DNA microarray. Proceedings of the National Academy of Sciences of the United States of America. 2001 Aug;**98**(17):9819-9823

[13] Ho SP, Bao Y, Lesher T, Malhotra R, Ma LY, Fluharty SJ, et al. Mapping of RNA accessible sites for antisense experiments with oligonucleotide libraries. Nature Biotechnology. 1998 Jan;**16**(1):59-63

[14] Andronescu M, Zhang ZC, Condon A. Secondary structure prediction of interacting RNA molecules. Journal of Molecular Biology. 2005 Feb;**345**(5):987-1001

[15] Vickers TA, Wyatt JR, Freier SM. Effects of RNA secondary structure on cellular antisense activity. Nucleic Acids Research. 2000 Mar;**28**(6):1340-1347

[16] Ding Y, Lawrence CE. Statistical prediction of single-stranded regions in RNA secondary structure and application to predicting effective antisense target sites and beyond.

Nucleic Acids Research. 2001 Mar;**29**(5):1034-1046

[17] Far RK, Nedbal W, Sczakiel G. Concepts to automate the theoretical design of effective antisense oligonucleotides. Bioinformatics. 2001 Nov;**17**(11):1058-1061

[18] Yang SP, Song ST, Tang ZM, Song HF. Optimization of antisense drug design against conservative local motif in simulant secondary structures of HER-2 mRNA and QSAR analysis. Acta Pharmacologica Sinica. 2003 Sep;**24**(9):897-902

[19] Matveeva OV, Tsodikov AD, Giddings M, Freier SM, Wyatt JR, Spiridonov AN, et al. Identification of sequence motifs in oligonucleotides whose presence is correlated with antisense activity. Nucleic Acids Research. 2000 Aug;**28**(15):2862-2865

[20] Deleavey GF, Damha MJ. Designing chemically modified oligonucleotides for targeted gene silencing. Chemistry & Biology. 2012 Aug;**19**(8):937-954

[21] Juliano RL, Ming X, Nakagawa O. The chemistry and biology of oligonucleotide conjugates. Accounts of Chemical Research. 2012 Jul;**45**(7):1067-1076

[22] Juliano RL. The delivery of therapeutic oligonucleotides. Nucleic Acids Research. 2016 Aug;**44**(14):6518-6548

[23] Eckstein F. Phosphorothioates, essential components of therapeutic oligonucleotides. Nucleic Acid Therapeutics. 2014 Dec;**24**(6):374-387

[24] Vitravene Study Group. A randomized controlled clinical trial of intravitreous fomivirsen for treatment of newly diagnosed peripheral cytomegalovirus retinitis in patients with AIDS. American Journal of Ophthalmology. 2002 Apr;**133**(4):467-474

[25] Yu RZ, Lemonidis KM, Graham MJ, Matson JE, Crooke RM, Tribble DL, et al. Cross-species comparison of in vivo PK/PD relationships for second-generation antisense oligonucleotides targeting apolipoprotein B-100. Biochemical Pharmacology. 2009 Mar;**77**(5):910-919

[26] Miyake A, Murata Y, Okazawa H, Ikeda H, Niwayama Y, Ohnishi H, et al. Negative regulation by SHPS-1 of toll-like receptor-dependent proinflammatory cytokine production in macrophages. Genes to Cells. 2008 Feb;**13**(2):209-219

[27] Winkler J, Stessl M, Amartey J, Noe CR. Off-target effects related to the phosphorothioate modification of nucleic acids. ChemMedChem. 2010 Aug;**5**(8):1344-1352

[28] Prakash TP, Kawasaki AM, Wancewicz EV, Shen L, Monia BP, Ross BS, et al. Comparing in vitro and in vivo activity of 2'-O-[2-(methylamino)-2-oxoethyl]- and 2'-O-methoxyethyl-modified antisense oligonucleotides. Journal of Medicinal Chemistry. 2008 May;**51**(9):2766-2776

[29] Kurreck J, Wyszko E, Gillen C, Erdmann VA. Design of antisense oligonucleotides stabilized by locked nucleic acids. Nucleic Acids Research. 2002 May;**30**(9):1911-1918

[30] Sioud M. Targeted delivery of antisense oligonucleotides and siRNAs into mammalian cells. Methods in Molecular Biology. 2009;**487**:61-82

[31] Crooke ST. Progress in antisense technology. Annual Review of Medicine. 2004;**55**:61-95

[32] Zamaratski E, Pradeepkumar PI, Chattopadhyaya J. A critical survey of the structure-function of the antisense oligo/RNA heteroduplex as substrate for RNase H. Journal of Biochemical and Biophysical Methods. 2001 May;**48**(3):189-208

[33] Yamamoto T, Nakatani M, Narukawa K, Obika S. Antisense drug discovery and development. Future Medicinal Chemistry. 2011 Mar;**3**(3):339-365

[34] Gleave ME, Monia BP. Antisense therapy for cancer. Nature Reviews. Cancer. 2005 Jun;**5**(6):468-479

[35] Kurreck J. Antisense technologies. Improvement through novel chemical modifications. European Journal of Biochemistry. 2003 Apr;**270**(8):1628-1644

[36] Nielsen PE. PNA technology. Molecular Biotechnology. 2004 Mar;**26**(3):233-248

[37] Braasch DA, Corey DR. Novel antisense and peptide nucleic acid strategies for controlling gene expression. Biochemistry. 2002 Apr;**41**(14):4503-4510

[38] Nielsen PE. Antisense properties of peptide nucleic acid. Methods in Enzymology. 2000;**313**:156-164

[39] Koppelhus U, Nielsen PE. Cellular delivery of peptide nucleic acid (PNA). Advanced Drug Delivery Reviews. 2003 Feb;**55**(2):267-280

[40] Paulasova P, Pellestor F. The peptide nucleic acids (PNAs): A new generation of probes for genetic and cytogenetic analyses. Annales de Génétique. 2004 Oct-Dec;**47**(4):349-358

[41] Amantana A, Iversen PL. Pharmacokinetics and biodistribution of phosphorodiamidate morpholino antisense oligomers. Current Opinion in Pharmacology. 2005 Oct;**5**(5):550-555

[42] Seth PP, Siwkowski A, Allerson CR, Vasquez G, Lee S, Prakash TP, et al. Short antisense oligonucleotides with novel 2′-4′ conformationaly restricted nucleoside analogues show improved potency without increased toxicity in animals. Journal of Medicinal Chemistry. 2009 Jan;**52**(1):10-13

[43] Nelson MH, Stein DA, Kroeker AD, Hatlevig SA, Iversen PL, Moulton HM. Arginine-rich peptide conjugation to morpholino oligomers: Effects on antisense activity and specificity. Bioconjugate Chemistry. 2005 Jul-Aug;**16**(4):959-966

[44] Iversen PL, Arora V, Acker AJ, Mason DH, Devi GR. Efficacy of antisense morpholino oligomer targeted to c-myc in prostate cancer xenograft murine model and a phase I safety study in humans. Clinical Cancer Research. 2003 Jul;**9**(7):2510-2519

[45] Moulton JD, Jiang S. Gene knockdowns in adult animals: PPMOs and vivo-morpholinos. Molecules. 2009;**14**(3):1304-1323

[46] Fluiter K, Mook OR, Baas F. The therapeutic potential of LNA-modified siRNAs: Reduction of off-target effects by chemical modification of the siRNA sequence. Methods in Molecular Biology. 2009;**487**:189-203

[47] Vester B, Wengel J. LNA (locked nucleic acid): High-affinity targeting of complementary RNA and DNA. Biochemistry. 2004 Oct;**43**(42):13233-13241

[48] Bondensgaard K, Petersen M, Singh SK, Rajwanshi VK, Kumar R, Wengel J, et al. Structural studies of LNA:RNA duplexes by NMR: Conformations and implications for RNase H activity. Chemistry. 2000 Aug;**6**(15):2687-2695

[49] Fluiter K, Frieden M, Vreijling J, Rosenbohm C, De Wissel MB, Christensen SM, et al. On the in vitro and in vivo properties of four locked nucleic acid nucleotides incorporated into an anti-H-Ras antisense oligonucleotide. Chembiochem. 2005 Jun;**6**(6):1104-1109

[50] Petersen M, Wengel J. LNA: A versatile tool for therapeutics and genomics. Trends in Biotechnology. 2003 Feb;**21**(2):74-81

[51] Simoes-Wust AP, Hopkins-Donaldson S, Sigrist B, Belyanskaya L, Stahel RA, Zangemeister-Wittke U. A functionally improved locked nucleic acid antisense oligonucleotide inhibits Bcl-2 and Bcl-xL expression and facilitates tumor cell apoptosis. Oligonucleotides. 2004;**14**(3):199-209

[52] Dirin M, Winkler J. Influence of diverse chemical modifications on the ADME characteristics and toxicology of antisense oligonucleotides. Expert Opinion on Biological Therapy. 2013 Jun;**13**(6):875-888

[53] Koller E, Vincent TM, Chappell A, De S, Manoharan M, Bennett CF. Mechanisms of single-stranded phosphorothioate modified antisense oligonucleotide accumulation in hepatocytes. Nucleic Acids Research. 2011 Jun;**39**(11):4795-4807

[54] Gomes-da-Silva LC, Fonseca NA, Moura V, Pedroso de Lima MC, Simoes S, Moreira JN. Lipid-based nanoparticles for siRNA delivery in cancer therapy: Paradigms and challenges. Accounts of Chemical Research. 2012 Jul;**45**(7):1163-1171

[55] Geary RS, Watanabe TA, Truong L, Freier S, Lesnik EA, Sioufi NB, et al. Pharmacokinetic properties of 2'-O-(2-methoxyethyl)-modified oligonucleotide analogs in rats. The Journal of Pharmacology and Experimental Therapeutics. 2001 Mar;**296**(3):890-897

[56] Yu RZ, Zhang H, Geary RS, Graham M, Masarjian L, Lemonidis K, et al. Pharmacokinetics and pharmacodynamics of an antisense phosphorothioate oligonucleotide targeting Fas mRNA in mice. The Journal of Pharmacology and Experimental Therapeutics. 2001 Feb;**296**(2):388-395

[57] Butler M, Crooke RM, Graham MJ, Lemonidis KM, Lougheed M, Murray SF, et al. Phosphorothioate oligodeoxynucleotides distribute similarly in class a scavenger receptor knockout and wild-type mice. The Journal of Pharmacology and Experimental Therapeutics. 2000 Feb;**292**(2):489-496

[58] McMahon BM, Mays D, Lipsky J, Stewart JA, Fauq A, Richelson E. Pharmacokinetics and tissue distribution of a peptide nucleic acid after intravenous administration. Antisense & Nucleic Acid Drug Development. 2002 Apr;**12**(2):65-70

[59] Jason TL, Koropatnick J, Berg RW. Toxicology of antisense therapeutics. Toxicology and Applied Pharmacology. 2004 Nov;**201**(1):66-83

[60] Hanagata N. Structure-dependent immunostimulatory effect of CpG oligodeoxynucleotides and their delivery system. International Journal of Nanomedicine. 2012;**7**:2181-2195

[61] Vollmer J, Jepsen JS, Uhlmann E, Schetter C, Jurk M, Wader T, et al. Modulation of CpG oligodeoxynucleotide-mediated immune stimulation by locked nucleic acid (LNA). Oligonucleotides. 2004 Spring;**14**(1):23-31

[62] Sewell KL, Geary RS, Baker BF, Glover JM, Mant TG, Yu RZ, et al. Phase I trial of ISIS 104838, a 2′-methoxyethyl modified antisense oligonucleotide targeting tumor necrosis factor-alpha. The Journal of Pharmacology and Experimental Therapeutics. 2002 Dec;**303**(3):1334-1343

[63] Uhlmann E, Vollmer J. Recent advances in the development of immunostimulatory oligonucleotides. Current Opinion in Drug Discovery & Development. 2003 Mar;**6**(2):204-217

[64] Islam A, Handley SL, Thompson KS, Akhtar S. Studies on uptake, sub-cellular trafficking and efflux of antisense oligodeoxynucleotides in glioma cells using self-assembling cationic lipoplexes as delivery systems. Journal of Drug Targeting. 2000;**7**(5):373-382

[65] Li J, Chen YC, Tseng YC, Mozumdar S, Huang L. Biodegradable calcium phosphate nanoparticle with lipid coating for systemic siRNA delivery. Journal of Controlled Release. 2010 Mar;**142**(3):416-421

[66] Tseng YC, Mozumdar S, Huang L. Lipid-based systemic delivery of siRNA. Advanced Drug Delivery Reviews. 2009 Jul;**61**(9):721-731

[67] Kang H, Alam MR, Dixit V, Fisher M, Juliano RL. Cellular delivery and biological activity of antisense oligonucleotides conjugated to a targeted protein carrier. Bioconjugate Chemistry. 2008 Nov;**19**(11):2182-2188

[68] Lysik MA, Wu-Pong S. Innovations in oligonucleotide drug delivery. Journal of Pharmaceutical Sciences. 2003 Aug;**92**(8):1559-1573

[69] Benimetskaya L, Guzzo-Pernell N, Liu ST, Lai JC, Miller P, Stein CA. Protamine-fragment peptides fused to an SV40 nuclear localization signal deliver oligonucleotides that produce antisense effects in prostate and bladder carcinoma cells. Bioconjugate Chemistry. 2002 Mar-Apr;**13**(2):177-187

[70] Jarver P, Langel U. The use of cell-penetrating peptides as a tool for gene regulation. Drug Discovery Today. 2004 May;**9**(9):395-402

[71] Kaihatsu K, Huffman KE, Corey DR. Intracellular uptake and inhibition of gene expression by PNAs and PNA-peptide conjugates. Biochemistry. 2004 Nov;**43**(45):14340-14347

[72] Shabanpoor F, McClorey G, Saleh AF, Jarver P, Wood MJ, Gait MJ. Bi-specific splice-switching PMO oligonucleotides conjugated via a single peptide active in a mouse model of Duchenne muscular dystrophy. Nucleic Acids Research. 2015 Jan;**43**(1):29-39

[73] Stockert RJ. The asialoglycoprotein receptor: Relationships between structure, function, and expression. Physiological Reviews. 1995 Jul;**75**(3):591-609

[74] Steirer LM, Park EI, Townsend RR, Baenziger JU. The asialoglycoprotein receptor regulates levels of plasma glycoproteins terminating with sialic acid alpha2,6-galactose. The Journal of Biological Chemistry. 2009 Feb;**284**(6):3777-3783

[75] Baenziger JU, Maynard Y. Human hepatic lectin. Physiochemical properties and specificity. The Journal of Biological Chemistry. 1980 May;**255**(10):4607-4613

[76] Nair JK, Willoughby JL, Chan A, Charisse K, Alam MR, Wang Q, et al. Multivalent N-acetylgalactosamine-conjugated siRNA localizes in hepatocytes and elicits robust RNAi-mediated gene silencing. Journal of the American Chemical Society. 2014 Dec;**136**(49):16958-16961

[77] Prakash TP, Graham MJ, Yu J, Carty R, Low A, Chappell A, et al. Targeted delivery of antisense oligonucleotides to hepatocytes using triantennary N-acetyl galactosamine improves potency 10-fold in mice. Nucleic Acids Research. 2014 Jul;**42**(13):8796-8807

[78] Liu Y, Bergan R. Improved intracellular delivery of oligonucleotides by square wave electroporation. Antisense & Nucleic Acid Drug Development. 2001 Feb;**11**(1):7-14

[79] Karaki S, Benizri S, Mejias R, Baylot V, Branger N, Nguyen T, et al. Lipid-oligonucleotide conjugates improve cellular uptake and efficiency of TCTP-antisense in castration-resistant prostate cancer. Journal of Controlled Release. 2017 Jul;**258**:1-9

Chapter 3

MiRNA-Based Therapeutics in Oncology, Realities, and Challenges

Ovidiu Balacescu, Simona Visan, Oana Baldasici, Loredana Balacescu, Catalin Vlad and Patriciu Achimas-Cadariu

Abstract

As master modulators of the human genome, miRNAs are involved in all cancer hallmarks, disrupting the normal function of their targets. By gaining or losing the function, miRNAs lead to the validation of tumor phenotype, its progression, and metastasis as well as to drug resistance. Increasing the evidence suggests that the modulation of miRNAs in cancer cells, by suppressing the oncogenic miRNAs (oncomiRs) and substituting the deficient tumor suppressive miRNAs (TS-miRNAs), could become a reliable tool for improving the cancer therapy. In this chapter, we will present an up-to-date overview of the role of miRNA-based therapeutics in oncology, highlighting their role in cancer management, how these therapies can be used, and which would be the future challenges related to miRNA-based therapies.

Keywords: cancer, invasions, metastasis, miRNA, therapy

1. Introduction

With an increasing incidence each year, cancer represents a major health problem worldwide, ranked second, after cardiovascular disease. According to the last estimation presented by the International Agency for Research on Cancer (IARC) in 2012, more than 14 million new cases of cancers were encountered, while the cancer-related deaths reached around 8.2 million people [1]. Unfortunately, the estimation for 2030 shows an increase in over 21 million new cancer cases and about 13 million cancer deaths [2]. Cancer is characterized by changing the phenotype of the cells in which it occurs, leading to an uncontrolled proliferation, invasion, and metastasis. Albeit the cancers in early stages are treatable, especially by surgery, the major challenge is to treat cancers in advanced stages. Currently, the therapeutic regimens for treating the advanced cancers depend on several factors such as localization, phenotype, and tumor size and are based on a combination of at least two of more approaches, represented by surgery, chemotherapy, radiotherapy, hormone therapy, and target therapy. Nevertheless, this anticancer armamentarium is not very efficient because about 90% of advanced cancers lead to metastasis and death ultimately [3]. Current anticancer therapies target either antiproliferative or pro-apoptotic pathways of tumor cells or activate immune response against tumors, but

IntechOpen

none of the currently available antitumor therapies target the molecular pathways involved in invasion and metastasis.

Tumor invasion and metastasis, as they were pointed out by Hanahan and Weinberg [4], represent one of the most important hallmarks of cancer, and therefore, exploiting these features of tumor cells could bring new data to develop more powerful anticancer therapies. Tumor invasion and metastasis are very complex processes that involve a series of sequential and interrelated steps. In this line, epithelial-to-mesenchymal transition (EMT) represents the most important event underlying the tumor invasion [5]. During EMT, tumor cells lose their epithelial characteristics and adhesion and acquire increased motility by shifting toward a mesenchymal phenotype while also diminishing apoptosis and senescence and gaining stem cell properties. The EMT regulation includes a network of many regulators, inducers, and effector molecules, which sustains tumor cell dissemination to distant organs [6].

The "omics" revolution has brought us new data about the complexity of signaling pathways in cancer, the type of molecules that are involved in them, and which alterations are associated with cancer. Moreover, noncoding RNAs, including miRNAs, have proved their crucial role in the regulation of mRNA translation in both physiological and pathological status. Because of their high capacity to modulate mRNA expression, miRNAs are defined as master modulators of the human genome. Therefore, miRNAs are involved in all cancer hallmarks, disrupting the normal function of their targets. By gaining or losing the function, miRNAs lead to the validation of tumor phenotype, its progression, and metastasis as well as to drug resistance.

Increasing the evidence suggests that the modulation of miRNA expression in cancer cells, through the inhibition of oncogenic miRNAs (oncomiRs) and the substitution of deficient tumor suppressive miRNAs (TS-miRNAs), could represent a reliable tool for improving the cancer therapy. In this chapter, we will present an up-to-date overview about the role of miRNA-based therapeutics in oncology, highlighting their role in cancer management, how these therapies can be used, and which would be the future challenges related to miRNA-based therapies.

2. Short overview about biogenesis and function of miRNAs

If deciphering the whole human genome has represented a milestone of modern biology, the identification of its precise functionality is still a great challenge. However, by completing the ENCODE project, many data about how the human genome is functioning were revealed. Such as, it is estimated that about 1.5% of human genome includes coding DNA exons from protein-coding genes (PCGs), while the rest of 98% represents noncoding DNAs including regulatory sequences such as the ones defining noncoding RNAs (ncRNAs), as well as introns, and other DNA sequences with unknown functions [7].

About 80% of human genome is activated in cell physiology, and an important part of noncoding regulatory elements involved in the regulation of PCGs includes noncoding RNAs. Since their recognition as a distinct class of biological regulators [8], micro-RNAs (miRNAs) have become the most studied species of noncoding RNAs. miRNAs are coded by genes located in almost all regions of the genome, including both PCGs and noncoding transcripts. About a half of miRNA genes are located in both intronic (40%) and exonic (10%) regions of noncoding genes, while the majority of the other miRNA loci are located in intragenic regions of PCGs [9]. The first step of miRNA biogenesis includes the transcription of pri-miRNA, a primary long hairpin transcript with a length of hundreds or thousands of nucleotides (**Figure 1**). Furthermore, after its processing to a shorter

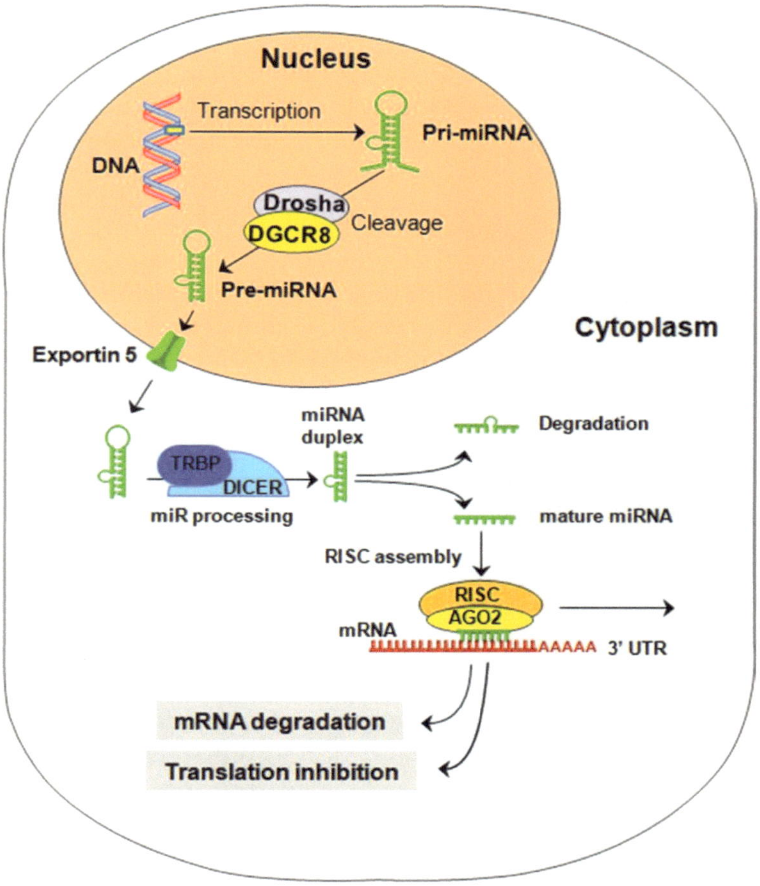

Figure 1.
miRNA biogenesis. The miRNA biogenesis starts in the nucleus, with a pri-miRNA transcription. Afterward, the pri-miRNA is processed to a shorter hairpin structure of about 70 nucleotides, by Drosha and DGCR8, and it is exported in the cytoplasm by Exportin 5. After enzymatic processing by DICER, double-stranded miRNAs are reduced to a single-stranded mature RNA (21–23 nucleotides in length). Furthermore, by incorporating into Argonaute 2 and RISC, mature miRNA will target mRNA transcripts, usually in the 3′ UTR, leading to mRNA degradation or repression.

hairpin structure of about 70 nucleotides, the pre-miRNA is exported into the cytoplasm, where under enzymatic processing, it is reduced to a single-stranded RNA (mature miRNA) of about 21–23 nucleotides in length. Afterward, by its incorporation into Argonaute 2 protein and then in the RNA-induced silencing complex (RISC), the mature miRNA will function as a guide molecule for silencing complex, targeting specific mRNA transcripts, usually by base-pairing specific mRNA transcripts, in the 3′ untranslated region (3′ UTR). Targeting the mRNA by a specific miRNA leads to the translational repression of mRNA and its exonucleolytic decay [9].

Because of their capacity to modulate up to 60% of PCGs, miRNAs are defined as "master modulators" of the human genome [10]. An important feature of miRNAs is that a single miRNA can target up to 200 mRNAs, while a single mRNA can be modulated by different miRNAs [11]. Nevertheless, to increase the accuracy of miRNA-mRNA binding, several combinatorial prediction tools based on thermodynamic modeling and machine learning techniques have been developed lately [12, 13], bringing new understanding about how miRNAs can exert their regulatory function through a combinatorial-cooperative activity.

At the moment, 48,885 mature miRNA products from 271 species, including 2654 mature human miRNAs, have been reported in the latest available miRNA database (miRBase release 22; http://www.mirbase.org/) [14]. In normal phenotype, by their modulatory effects, miRNAs maintain the cell physiology, while by their aberrant expression, miRNAs lead to the validation of many diseases including cancer.

3. The role of miRNAs in cancer

Croce's group established for the first time an association of mRNAs with cancer, indicating an alteration of miR-15a/16-1 cluster, in chronic lymphocytic leukemia [15]. Further functional analyses have demonstrated that miR-15 and miR-16 can target and suppress the expression of BCL2 oncogene, inducing the apoptosis. [16]. Through exploring the role of miRNAs, Croce's group has demonstrated that miRNA profiling could be taken into consideration for characterizing the malignant phenotype [17], opening a new perspective for identifying new cancer-specific miRNAs. Interestingly, for poorly differentiated tumors, tissue miRNA profiling has revealed better diagnosis than mRNA profiling, highlighting their role as tumor biomarkers [18]. An important feature of miRNAs, given by their high stability in formalin-fixed paraffin embedded (FFPE) tissues, blood including serum and plasma, as well as other biological fluids such as urine, tears, breast milk, saliva, and seminal fluids, makes them important candidates for the discovery of new minimally invasive biomarkers [19, 20]

Therefore, a myriad of studies describing the role of miRNAs in cancer development have been provided, with more than 21,565 papers that are published in PubMed today, when "miRNA, miR, microRNA, and cancer" are used as a string search.

Alteration of miRNA expression in cancer is due to genetic and epigenetic events. Genetic alterations include: chromosomal rearrangements or loss of heterozygosis (LOH) (e.g. miR-15a/16-1), gene amplification (e.g. miR-17-92 cluster, miR-155), deletions (e.g. let-7 family member), or mutations (e.g. miR-16) [15]. Moreover, genetic alteration may occur in the PCGs involved in the synthesis of the protein components of the Drosha, DGCR8, Exportin 5, Dicer, and AGO2, the main enzymes that process the biogenesis and activation of miRNAs. Pre- and post-transcriptional controls of not only miRNA biogenesis but also epigenetic events, including methylation and acetylation, were also related to aberrant expression of tumor miRNAs [21, 22]. Not lastly, the presence of the single-nucleotide polymorphism (SNP) mutations in the miRNA-coding genes may lead to the alterations of mature miRNA structure, reducing its specificity to the mRNA target [23].

Functionality studies have demonstrated that the expression of oncogenes and tumor-suppressor genes in cancer is closely controlled by miRNAs (**Figure 2**). Such as, miRNAs that target and modulate the oncogenic expression are defined as tumor-suppressor miRNAs (TS-miRNAs), while the miRNAs that modulate the expression of tumor-suppressor genes are known as oncomiRs [24]. Genetic and epigenetic alterations occurring in cancer lead to "gain of function" of oncomiRs and inactivation or "loss of function" of TS-miR (**Figure 2**), which translate into regulating the expression of their targets through downregulation of tumor-suppressor genes and upregulation of oncogenes, respectively [25]. miRNAs are involved in all hallmarks of cancer, including self-sufficiency in growth signals (let-7 family, miR-21), insensitivity to antigrowth signals (e.g. miR-17-92 cluster, miR-195), evasion from apoptosis (e.g. miR-34a, miR-185, miR-15/miR-16), limitless replicative potential (e.g. miR-372/373 cluster, miR221/222), angiogenesis (e.g. miR-210, miR-26, miR-15b, miR-155), invasion and metastases (e.g. miR-10b, miR-31, miR-200 family, miR-21, miR-15b), reprogramming energy metabolism

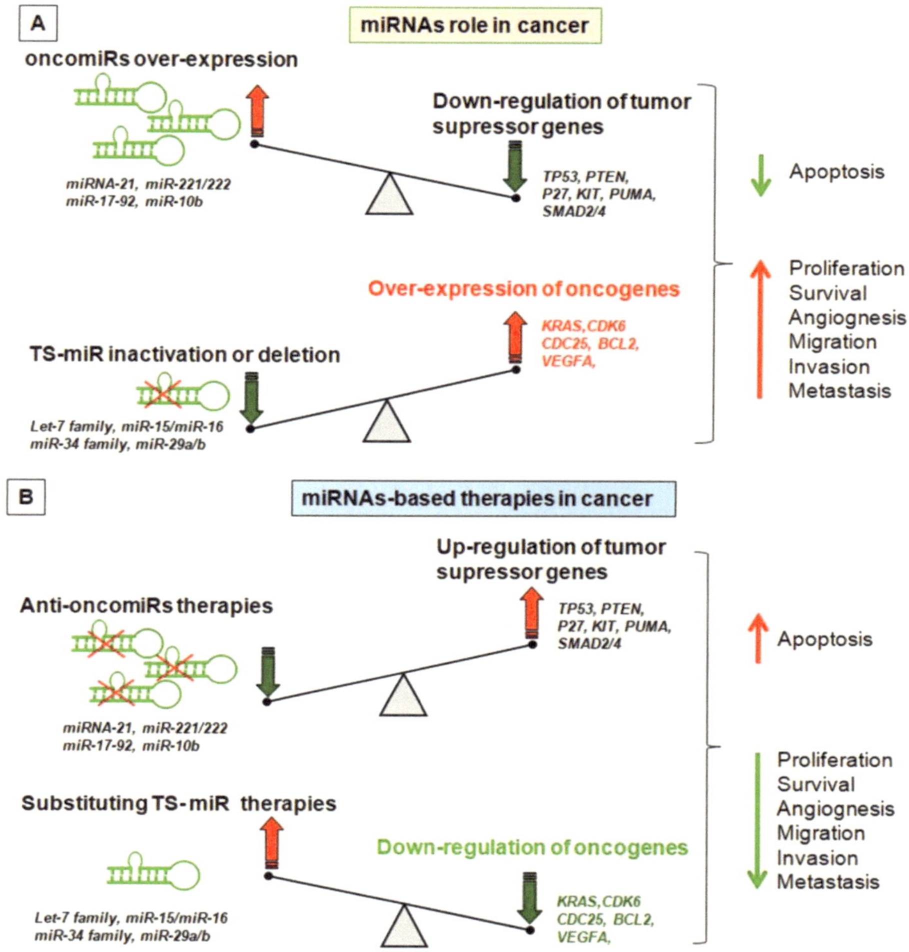

Figure 2.
The role of miRNAs in cancer and their use of miRNA-based therapy. **(A)** *miRNAs that function as oncomiRs and TS-miRs. Tumors are characterized by aberrant upregulation of oncomiRs that lead to downregulation of tumor-suppressor genes and inactivation of TS-miRs reflected in overexpression of oncogenes. All of these contribute to tumor development, invasion, and metastasis as well as decrease cell death.* **(B)** *The use of anti-miRNA therapies leads to block the oncomiR activities, resulting in the upregulation of tumor-suppressor genes, while substituting TS-miR therapies increases the cellular level of TS-miRs, leading to the inactivation of oncogenes. The effects of miRNA-based therapy indicate an increase in cell death concomitantly with inactivation of tumor development.*

(e.g. miR-23a/b, miR-378, miR-143, miR-15b), evading immune destruction (e.g. miR-124, miR-155, miR-17-92), tumor-promoting inflammation (miR-23b, miR-155, let-7d), and genomic instability (miR-21, miR-155, miR15b) [22, 26, 27].

4. Strategies used for miRNA-based therapies

4.1 miRNA inhibition therapies for oncomiRs

The choice to use mRNA-based therapies is based on the fact that the expression of mRNAs in tumor cells is altered, and tumor phenotype can be changed by the modulation of the miRNA expression [28].

MiRNA inhibition therapy is used to suppress the expression of oncomiRs that are frequently overexpressed in human cancers and reestablish the normal expression of tumor-suppressor genes that are targeting directly (**Figure 2**). The therapy for miRNA inhibition includes the following agents: antisense anti-miR oligonucleotides (AMOs), locked nucleic acid (LNA) anti-miRs, antagomiRs, miRNA sponges, and small molecule inhibitors of miRNAs (SMIRs) [27]. The principle of this therapy consists of an isolation of the endogenous miRNAs in an unrecognizable configuration, leading to inactivating and excluding the mature miRNAs from the RISC.

AMOs are single-stranded, chemically modified antisense oligonucleotides of about 17–22 nucleotides that are complementary to a miRNA of interest [28]. These antisense oligonucleotides anneal to the complementary mature miRNAs and inhibit their interaction with specific mRNA targets.

LNA anti-miRs represent an example of a modified antisense anti-miR oligonucleotide [29]. LNA-modified oligonucleotides present a higher thermal stability and affinity for their miRNA target molecules, as well as a higher aqueous solubility and increased metabolic stability for *in vivo* delivery [30].

The antagomiRs are single-stranded RNA molecules of about 23 nucleotides in length complementary to miRNA targets that are chemically modified to increase the stability of the RNA and protect it from degradation [31]. One of the most important aspects of using these agents is due to their lack of inducing any immune response.

miRNA sponges represent a class of RNAs that include multiple artificial binding sites similar to those found in the endogenous miRNA targets. The expression vectors represent the source of miRNA sponge transcription, thus reducing the miRNA's effects and increasing the expression of the miRNA's native targets [32].

SMIRs are small molecules that suppress the miRNA biogenesis or block the interaction between a miRNA and the target. The inhibition therapy using SMIRs is an encouraging one due to the reduced time of production, approval, and cost [33].

4.1.1 Discussion

Krützfeldt et al. [31] demonstrated that intravenous administration of several antagomiRs toward miR-16, miR-122, miR-192, and miR-194 leads to a significant reduction in the corresponding endogenous miRNAs.

Moreover, an important positive effect observed in this study was that after the administration of antagomiR-122, the cholesterol levels in plasma have decreased. Due to the fact that, so far, the therapy using antagomiRs did not induce a significant immune response, it is worth into consideration the development of a promising antisense therapy based on antagomiRs.

One of the main advantages of using locked nucleic acid (LNA) anti-miRs is that they present a higher thermal stability, high-affinity Watson-Crick hybridization with their RNA target molecules, higher aqueous solubility, and increased metabolic stability for *in vivo* delivery. Overexpression of miR-21 is a common place in glioblastomas, and Griveau et al.'s [34] study was able to silence miR-21 in U87MG glioblastoma cell line, using a LNA conjugated to lipid nanocapsules (LNC). Another advantage of using LNA-LNC complexes in combination with external beam radiation is represented by the improvement of cell sensitivity to treatment.

4.2 miRNA replacement therapies for tumor-suppressor miRNAs

Also defined as miRNA restoration therapy, the replacement therapy with miRNAs includes the following agents: small molecules, synthetic miRNA mimics, and DNA plasmids encoding a miRNA gene that epigenetically alters endogenous expression of miRNAs [35].

Small molecules in miRNA replacement therapy are represented by hypomethylating agents (Decitabine or 5-azacytidine) and enoxacin, exerting a role in the nonspecific miRNA expression.

miRNA mimics are double-stranded synthetic RNAs, which are aimed to compensate the lack of tumor-suppressor miRNAs by replacing the lost miRNAs. These chemically structures are loaded into RISC to provide the downstream inhibition of the target mRNAs [27].

4.2.1 Discussion

One of the main challenges of miRNA replacement therapy is represented by finding the most suitable, efficient, and specific delivery system. The efficacy of this therapy is significantly decreased by an unsuitable size of the vector or by gene expression. Since miRNAs can be introduced into cells using a similar technique to small interference RNAs [36], it is recommended to improve those techniques based on the insertion of synthetic miRNA mimics, DNA plasmids, and small molecules, as well as to improve the quality of molecules used for this type of therapy.

4.3 miRNA delivery systems

An important aspect that is worth considering in miRNA cancer therapy aims to use miRNA delivery systems. One of these delivery systems including microvesicles and exosomes aim to block miRNA-entrapped exosomes released by tumors. It is already demonstrated that miRNA-entrapped exosomes secreted by tumor cells can regulate gene expression in the receiving cells by binding to their target mRNAs [37]. The use of some agents that block specific miRNAs (such as LNA anti-miR-21 and LNA anti-miR-29a) in tumor cells could lead to the reduction in miRNA-entrapped exosomes, released by cancer cells [38]. However, an ideal delivery system meets the following criteria: protects the miRNAs from early degradation in the bloodstream, efficient distribution to the target cells, facilitates cellular uptake, does not induce an immune response, and made of biocompatible and biodegradable materials [39].

The most commonly used vectors for miRNA delivery include viral and nonviral vectors. Previous data demonstrated that viral vectors mainly caused an immune response; therefore, the focus of the actual studies is on developing efficient nonviral vectors. Nonviral vectors are classified into three main groups, including polymeric vectors (polyethyleneimines, atelocollagen, polylactic-co-glycolic acid, polyamidoamine dendrimers), lipid-based carriers (positively, negatively or neutral charged), and inorganic materials (gold, diamond, silica, and ferric oxide) [40].

The delivery system based on viral vectors transfers the pri-miRNA or mature miRNAs, usually a TS-miR, into a plasmid, which contains a viral promoter, an antibiotic resistance gene, and a restriction enzyme gene, to the tumor cells. After nuclear integration of the miRNA and further transcription, the mature miRNA represses the translation and/or induces the degradation of the target mRNA [41].

4.3.1 Discussion

One of the most studied classes of polymeric vectors was represented by polyethylenimines (PEIs) but was removed from clinical studies due to their high toxicity, given by an excessive positive charge, low biological degradation, and inactivation in serum caused by a nonspecific protein. Ibrahim et al. [42] have demonstrated that by using low molecular weight, PEIs as system delivery for miR-145 and miR-33a would decrease the toxicity and increase the antitumor effect, in a model of colon carcinoma. Recent studies [43, 44] have proved that codelivery of miR-200c with chitosan, a cationic polymer with a high specificity for nucleic acid binding, decreased the angiogenesis, invasion, EMT, and metastasis and increased the apoptosis, highlighting the role of miRNA concentration in treatment effectiveness. Hao et al. [45] used miRNA (MiR-15a, miR16-1)/ATE-APT complex formed by atelocollagen (ATE), a type I collagen positively charged polymer, in combination with a RNA aptamer (APT) used as a ligand to target PCa cells that express prostate-specific membrane antigen (PSMA). Their study concluded that miRNA/ATE-APT complex was more efficient than an ATE-miRNA complex and that by using a PSMA-targeted system, the chances for selective killing of prostate cancer cells significantly would increase.

Moreover, it is worth into consideration the administration methods used for synthetic miRNAs (miRNA mimics) delivery into cells. Previous studies of Trang et al. have shown that both intratumoral and intravenous administration of let-7a mimics lead to the diminishing of non-small-cell lung cancer (NSCLC) tumor size in mouse models [46, 47].

As a future improvement in miRNA delivery systems, it is recommended to be synthetized proteins or peptides in order to be used as vector polymeric due to their low cytotoxicity and immunogenicity. Finding a suitable delivery system for a specific miR according to tumor cell type and the development of systems to target specific cancer membrane antigens still represent major challenges.

5. MicroRNAs in cancer therapies

5.1 miRNA candidates used in preclinical trials

Increasing the evidence has demonstrated that miRNA expression is modified in cancer, and restoring the level of cellular miRNA could underpin the development of miRNA-based therapies. Below we briefly describe miRNAs that are currently used in preclinical and clinical trials and also represent examples that affect the emerging hallmarks of cancer such as evasion from apoptosis (miR-15/16, miR-34 cluster) [48], enabling replicative immortality (miR-34a) [48], activating invasion and metastasis (miR-10b) [49], tumor-promoting inflammation (miR-155), and genome instability and mutation (miR-155) [50].

5.1.1 miR-10b

Guessous et al. [51] observed that miR-10b is overexpressed in human glioblastoma and stem cell lines when compared to healthy tissues or astrocytes. After the modulation of miR-10b, they found out that the inhibition of miR-10b strongly reduced cell proliferation, invasion, and migration of glioblastoma and stem cell lines, whereas its overexpression caused cell migration and invasion. Moreover, in a previous study, Ma's group [52] has demonstrated that the use of miR-10b antagomiRs was correlated with reduced metastasis both in cell-culture lines and in animal model of breast tumor-bearing mice. Thus, miR-10b inhibition both *in vitro* and *in vivo* significantly decreased miR-10b levels and increased levels of Hoxd10 gene, an important miR-10b target. Curiously, the administration of miR-10b antagomiRs *in vivo* did not reduce primary mammary tumor growth but significantly suppressed the development of lung metastases, highlighting its antimetastatic role.

5.1.2 miR-221

Since miR-221 overexpression alters multiple cancer pathways, it becomes a potential target for miRNA-based therapy. In order to validate the role of miR-221 in tumorigenesis, Callegari et al.[53] showed that *in vivo* delivery of an AMO anti-miR-221 caused a significant decrease in the size and number of tumor nodules. Based on the results from their study, it was highlighted the promoter role of miR-221 in liver carcinogenesis, being also established a valuable animal model to investigate the anti-miRNA-based therapy for liver cancer.

Moreover, using a colorectal cancer model, Qin et al. [54] showed that miR-221 promotes cell migration and invasion *in vitro* and metastasis *in vivo,* identifying tumor-suppressor RECK gene as a direct target of miR-221.

With regard to the role of miR-221 in tumorigenesis combined with the need to limit its expression, Brognara's group demonstrated that a peptide nucleic acid conjugate targeted against miR-221 (Rpep-PNA-a221) caused a suppression of miR-221 expression and an upregulation of its target $p27^{Kip1}$ in two breast cancer cell lines (MCF-7 and MDA-MB-231), respectively [55]. On the other hand, in a recent study, Gallo et al. [56] evaluated the pharmacokinetic and pharmacodynamic properties of a locked nucleic acid anti-miR-221 (LNA-i-miR-221) in the models of mice and monkeys. Their data highlighted that LNA-anti-miR-221 has a short half-life, optimal tissue bioavailability and minimal urine excretion in both species. A very important aspect of their study was that no toxicity was present in the pilot monkey study. This finding defines the potential application of LNA-anti-miRNAs in clinical studies.

5.1.3 miR-222

Sometimes developing a miRNA-based therapy is difficult because the same miRNA can act both as an oncogene and as a tumor-suppressor gene, due to its multiple targets and mechanisms of action. Such an example in this way is represented by miR-222, which has a role of oncomiR in liver cancers, by targeting and suppressing the PTEN tumor-suppressor gene, or TS-miRNA, whose downregulation in erythroblastic leukemia leads to the overexpression of c-KIT oncogene [27].

5.1.4 miR-34

miR-34 is one of the most important TS-miRs, being positively controlled by TP53 [57], repressed by MYC [58], and silenced by aberrant CpG methylation [59].

Overexpression of miR-34 was related to apoptosis and cell cycle arrest [60], while its underexpression was linked to different tumor types, including nonsmall-cell lung cancer (NSCLC) [61], breast cancer [62], or ovarian cancer [63]. Several studies have proved that ionizing radiation upregulates the levels of expression from different miR-34 family members in a variety of human cell types: miR-34b in lymphocytes [64], miR-34c in prostate cancer cell lines [65], and miR-34a in thyroid cells [66]. Consequently, to increase the therapeutic efficiency, some of the future studies should focus on the combined use of DNA damage response related to miRNAs and radio- or chemotherapy. By performing a miR-34 modulation, Trang et al. [47] have demonstrated that synthetic miR-34 mimics incorporated in a lipid-based particle was able to block tumor growth in a mouse model of nonsmall cell lung. Likewise, Daige et al. [67] have proved that the use of encapsulating miR-34a mimics into liposomes (MRX34) leads to increase the level of miR34a in liver tumors, followed by significantly reducing several of its mRNA targets, and consequently tumor regression.

Based on these results, encapsulating miR-34a mimics into liposomes (MRX34, Mirna Therapeutics Inc.) was later proposed to be investigated in clinical trials [68].

5.1.5 miR-16

miR-16 represents another TS-miR whose decreased expression has been observed among different types of cancers, as well as in nonsmall cell lung cancer (NSCLC) [69], prostate cancer [70], or malignant pleural mesothelioma [71], making it a strong candidate for replacement therapy in future studies with potential use in clinical trials. The data presented by Takeshita et al. [72] revealed that systemic delivery of synthetic miR-16, conjugated to atelocollagen, significantly reduced bone metastases and tumor development in a prostate cancer animal model. Moreover, their *in vitro* data suggest that miR-16 suppresses prostate tumor growth by regulating the expression of genes associated with cell-cycle control and cellular proliferation such as CDK1 and CDK2. The Hao group has also revealed that miR-16-1/atelocollagen-aptamer complex used in a mice model of human prostate cancer with bone metastasis enhanced anticancer efficacy. They also demonstrated that the efficacy of this complex, including aptamers, was higher, both *in vitro* and *in vivo* models than the other atelocollagen complexes that do not include aptamers. Re-expression of miR-16 mimic in malignant pleural mesothelioma cell lines and nude mouse models has caused the inhibition of tumor growth, correlated with downregulation of target genes Bcl-2 and CCND1 [71].

5.1.6 miR-155

miR-155, one of the first described oncomiRs [73], was identified as highly expressed in a wide range of tumors including chronic lymphocytic leukemia [74], lung cancer [75], breast cancer [76], acute myeloid leukemia [77], solid tumor including stomach, prostate, colon, pancreas [78], and melanoma [79].

OncomiR-155 was discovered to target RAD51, an important gene in the homologous recombination DNA repair pathway, and the clinical study of Gasparini et al. [80] for triple negative breast cancer revealed that low miR-155 expression level correlated with worse progression-free survival. Moreover, Pouliot et al. [81] reported a reduced expression of miR-155 in human epidermoid carcinoma cisplatin-resistant cell lines. Dysregulated expression of this miRNA sensitizes the cells to cisplatin-induced apoptosis by targeting WEE1 and CHK1 kinases. Based on these results, future studies are encouraged with the focus on the use of exogenous agents, such as mimics or anti-miRs to sensitize cancer cells to chemo- or radiotherapy, thus overcoming resistance to therapy.

Alexander et al. [82] found that endogenous miR-155, an important microRNA that regulates inflammation, is released from dendritic cells within exosomes and transferred to recipient dendritic cells. Administration of miR-155 containing exosomes enhances inflammatory gene expression as a response to endotoxin-induced inflammation in mice. Their findings provide strong evidence that endogenous microRNAs follow a functional transfer between immune cells and represent a regulatory mechanism for inflammatory response.

More examples of tumor-suppressor miRNA mimics, which target multiple oncogenic transcripts, were recently presented by Hosseinahli et al. [41].

5.2 Clinical studies involving miRNA-based therapy

Given the results provided by *in vitro* and *in vivo* studies, several clinical trials including miRNA-based therapy in human cancers were subsequently initiated (**Table 1**).

Company	Drug	Targeted miRNA	Therapy type	Cancer type	Delivery system	Mechanism/effect	Trial status	Clinical trials. Gov identifier
Mirna Therapeutics. Inc	MRX34	miR-34	Mimic	Nonsmall-cell lung carcinoma, small cell lung cancer, primary liver cancer lymphoma, melanoma, multiple myeloma, renal cell carcinoma	LNPs (Smarticles)	Reduction in the expression of oncogenes, tumor regression, enhanced the survival, and inhibited the growth of other nonhepatic tumors	Multicenter phase I terminated	NCT01829971
EnGeneIC	MesomiR-1	miR-16	Mimic	Malignant pleural mesothelioma, nonsmall cell lung cancer	EnGeneIC delivery vehicle	Strong inhibition of tumor growth	Multicenter phase I completed	NCT02369198
miRagen Therapeutics	MRG-106	miR-155	Anti-miR	Cutaneous T cell lymphoma, mycosis fungoides, chronic lymphocytic leukemia, adult T-cell leukemia/lymphoma	LNA-modified antisense inhibitor	Reduce overexpression and of oncomiR, leading to decreasing aberrant cell proliferation	Multicenter phase I recruiting	NCT02580552

Table 1.
Clinical trials using miRNA therapy in human cancers (adapted after Christopher et al. [87] and Rupaimoole et al. [88]).

In April 2013, Mirna Therapeutics, Inc., a publicly traded company based in Carlsbad, California, which primarily focuses on anti-miRNAs technology, announced that their leading product candidate, MRX34, a mimic of miR-34 encapsulated in a liposomal nanoparticle formulation, called NOV40, was the first microRNA mimic to enter clinical development. The multicenter phase I trial of MRX34 included patients diagnosed with primary liver cancer, nonsmall cell lung cancer (NSCLC), lymphoma, melanoma, multiple myeloma, or renal cell carcinoma. The trial aimed to increase the number of intravenously doses with two times per week or five times per day schedule. In June 2016, a total of 99 patients suffering from HCC, NSCLC, or pancreatic cancer had been enrolled in the study [83]. The phase I clinical trial confirmed partial responses in a patient with metastasized hepatocellular carcinoma (HCC), a patient with advanced acral melanoma, and a patient with advanced renal cell carcinoma (RCC), evaluated through Response Evaluation Criteria in Solid Tumors (RECIST). Also, 14 patients were detected with stable disease (median duration 136 days; range 79–386 days). Results from white blood cell analysis indicated a significant reduction in two miR-34 target genes FOXP1 and BCL2. Nonetheless, because of the immune-related adverse responses involving patient deaths, the trial was finished. Since the cause of these immune reactions remains still unclear, preclinical trials will be need in order to better understand the immune-related toxicities. After passing successfully the phase I clinical trial, they intended to advance into two phase II clinical studies: one for patients diagnosed with advanced malignant melanoma and another for patients diagnosed with advanced renal cell carcinoma (RCC). In concordance with the advancements made by MRX34, their lead product candidate, through the clinical development, miR-34 mimics represent a new promising class of replacement therapy used in cancer. Additionally, Cortez et al. [84] reported that p53 regulated PDL1 expression via miR-34 in nonsmall-cell lung cancer. Administration of miR-34a mimics (MRX34), alone or in combination with radiotherapy (XRT), reduced PDL1 expression in the tumor and antagonized T-cell exhaustion.

In November 2014, EnGeneIC, a privately held Australian company in collaboration with Asbestos Diseases Research Institute, Sydney, Australia, announced the start of phase I clinical trial using miR-16 mimic charged in nanocells, a bacterial-derived transfection system EDV™. The trial included patients suffering from malignant pleural mesothelioma (MPM) and advanced nonsmall cell lung cancer (NSCLC), refractory to standard therapy. miR-16 mimic-based therapy were delivered intravenously, using EnGeneIC Delivery Vehicle (EDV)-Packaging, and were surface conjugated with an EGFR-targeting antibody in order to facilitate the target of tumor site [85]. Preliminary data presented by Van Zandwijk et al. [86] show manageable safety in response to infusion of 5 billion nanocells loaded with 1.5 μg miR-15/16 mimics as a first-dose level in the first five patients that had been enrolled. Because of the fact that this targomiR trial using miR-16 as a replacement therapy did not present adverse immune response and toxic effects, it is expected to continue to phase II study [86].

In March 2016, MiRagen Therapeutics, Inc., a privately held company based in Boulder, Colorado, announced the initiation of phase I clinical trial to investigate the anticancer product candidate: MRG-106, a synthetic microRNA antagonist of microRNA-155 (LNA anti-miR). The phase I clinical trial is currently tested in patients diagnosed with cutaneous T-cell lymphoma (CTCL) of the mycosis fungoides (MF) subtype [89].

Despite some promising preclinical results, the outcome of MRX34 translational clinical trial using miR-16 as a replacement therapy, designed to restore the expression of miR-34 in patients diagnosed with different types of cancer, was discouraging due to adverse toxic effects. At present, this clinical trial is finished, and its suitability to further development to phase II study remains under question.

However, this drawback can be addressed by optimizing therapeutic doses and applying organ-specific administration routes [41].

6. Future challenges: new reliable miRNAs for target therapies

Epithelial-to-mesenchymal transition (EMT) allows tumor cells to enter the metastatic cascade by changing their morphological and molecular characteristics, and it represents a wide spectrum that cancer cells keep transiting. The EMT program relies on an intricate network of signaling pathways that dictate a series of phenotypic changes in epithelial cells. One clearly visible aspect is the loss of apical-basal polarity and cell-to-cell interaction caused by the destabilization of tight junctions, decreased claudin, occludin, and E-cadherin repression by SNAIL, SLUG, ZEB, TWIST, and SMAD, and its interchange with N-cadherin, a process known as the "cadherin switch" [90, 91]. Moreover, the overexpression of vimentin, a cytoskeleton intermediate-filament protein of mesenchymal origin that connects the nucleus to the plasma membrane, enables filopodia formation and a fibroblastic spindle-like morphology. Vimentin was proved to be induced through Slug and Ras signaling, and it promotes cell movement and migration [92]. The next step is the degradation of extracellular matrix components under the activity of matrix metalloproteinases and the invasion of the surrounding stroma (**Figure 3**).

The EMT is coordinated by a series of signaling pathways triggered by either the tumor microenvironment or the intrinsic factors, and it falls under the incidence of regulatory noncoding RNAs, especially micro-RNAs [93].

This is the reason why finding potential microRNA targets for blocking EMT could support the efforts already made in blocking metastasis and improving cancer therapy strategies. Right below, we are succinctly reviewing the results of several studies that investigated the role of microRNAs in EMT and metastasis and their potential in becoming microRNA therapy targets (**Table 2**).

The influence of cancer-associated fibroblasts (CAFs) secreted exosomes over endometrial cancer progression was questioned in a study by Li et al. [94]. CAFs secreted exosomes contained significantly lower levels of miR-148b than normal fibroblasts, and miR-148b expression was lower in endometrial cancer specimens than in normal adjacent tissues. miR-148b was correlated with improved prognosis, *in vitro* and *in vivo* studies suggesting its role as an EMT inhibitor. Downregulation of DNMT1 oncogene was the mechanism proposed for miR-148b-mediated suppression of endometrial cancer progression. Also, relating to the tumor microenvironment, emerging evidence shows the prometastatic effect of a hypoxic

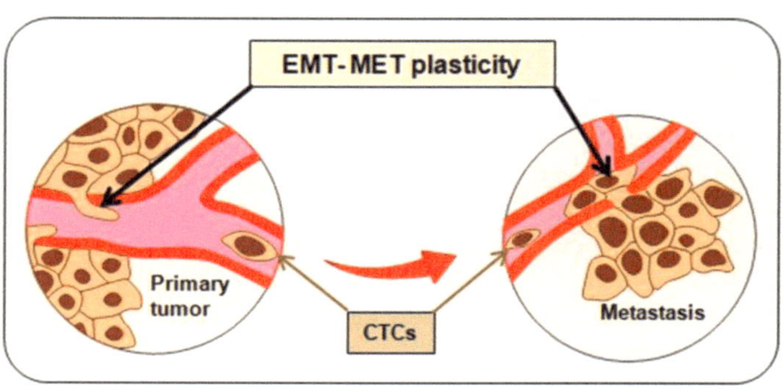

Figure 3.
The EMT-MET plasticity of tumor cells, their migration, and invasion as tumor circulating cells (CTCs).

microenvironment over tumor cells. Acidic conditions were shown to promote miR-210 overexpression by activating HIF1 [95, 96]. In prostate cancer, high levels of miR-210 were detected in bone metastases, and they were correlated with poor prognosis of prostate cancer patients. Exogenously overexpression of miR-210-3p in cancer cell lines enhanced cell motility and migration as well as bone metastasis in mouse model by inducing NF-κB signaling and EMT. Moreover, miR-210-3p inhibition reversed EMT and impaired the metastatic potential of cancer cells [95]. Another study confirmed the hypoxia-induced EMT activation and metastasis by HIF1-miR-210 axis in breast cancer. Tang et al. [96] identified high expression of miR-210 in hypoxia grown breast cancer stem cells and in isolated human breast cancer stem cells. The overexpression of MiR-210 in poorly metastatic MCF7 cell lines leads to their invasiveness and migration *in vitro* as well as increasing metastatic potential *in vivo*. One suggested mechanism is related to the direct binding of miR-210 to the Open Reading Frame (ORF) of the E-cadherin mRNA and its post-transcriptional inhibition in breast cancer cells.

miR-652 downregulation in the acidic microenvironment of pancreatic cancer promoted EMT by ZEB1 activation, and it was correlated with a progressive stage, lymphatic invasion, vascular infiltration, and distant metastasis. *In vitro* experiments showed that miR-652 overexpression has an antimetastatic effect by inducing MET in PANC-1-A miR-652-mimic transfected cells, and it reduced their migration and invasion. Also, *in vivo* studies confirmed the *in vitro* results with lower tumor mass, fewer metastases, and overexpression of E-cadherin over vimentin/N-cadherin in mouse xenografts PANC-1-A miR-652-mimic transfected cells vs. miR-652 inhibitor [97].

Partially due to cancer tumors heterogeneity in construction and behavior and the relative novelty of noncoding RNAs as potential targets for cancer therapy, there are still missing bricks in understanding the mechanism that triggers the regulation of cancer-related microRNAs. However, as shown above, tumor microenvironment has a great impact over cancer progression, and probably understanding its role in modulating microRNA expression in tumor cells might bring light to new potential targets for improved therapy.

From a different perspective, there are many well-known pathways underlying cancer development and progression. Wnt signaling pathway represents one of the fundamental pathways involved in cell proliferation and specialization, as well as cell movement during both embryonic development and tissue homeostasis. The canonical Wnt signaling functions by regulating the amount of the transcriptional coactivator β-catenin, a molecule that controls key developmental gene expression programs [98]. Wnt signaling aberrations have been shown to regulate various processes that are important for cancer progression, including tumor initiation, tumor growth, cell senescence, cell death, differentiation, and metastasis. Wnt signaling molecules and downstream effectors can promote transcriptional changes in order to induce EMT in cancer cells while also being further activated by EMT in a continuous feedback loop [99].

Several microRNAs were proven to modulate Wnt signaling in EMT and cancer metastasis. In endometrial cancer, Wnt signaling can be activated by miR-652, which targets and inhibits retinoid orphan nuclear receptor alpha (RORA) gene. RORA represents a tumor-suppressor gene that represses the Wnt/β-catenin pathway through attenuating β-catenin transcriptional activity. Expression of miR-652 is frequently increased in human endometrial cancer tissues, its high expression being correlated with poor tumor differentiation, shorter overall survival, and recurrence. Overexpression of miR-652 in endometrial cancer cell promotes their proliferation and migration *in vitro* and *in vivo* [100].

Another metastasis enhancer, miR-374a, acts by activating the Wnt/β-catenin cascade and promoting EMT. miR-374a maintains constitutively activated

Wnt/β-catenin signaling by suppressing multiple negative regulators including WIF1, PTEN, and WNT5A. miR-374a was upregulated in primary tumor samples from breast cancer patients with distant metastases, and it was associated with poor metastasis-free survival. miR-374a transfection into poorly metastatic MCF7 cell line promoted its motility and invasiveness *in vitro* and lung metastasis forming abilities in BALB/c mice, while miR-374a knockdown in highly invasive MDA-MB-231 cells decreased their motility and metastatic potential [101].

On the other hand, microRNA-590-5p was found to function as a tumor-suppressor in breast cancer, inhibiting EMT, cell migration, and invasion by downregulating the Wnt/β-catenin pathway. Quantitative RT-PCR analysis on breast tumor tissues and paired adjacent normal tissues showed that miR-590-5p was downregulated in breast cancer together with E-cadherin, while its target PITX2, b-catenin, Wnt-1, N-cadherin, and vimentin were upregulated. *In vitro* experiments and mouse xenografts showed that miR-590-5p upregulation or PITX2 silencing inhibits the activation of Wnt/β-catenin signaling pathway and suppresses the EMT of breast cancer [102].

Another metastasis inhibitor, miR-625, was characterized in different pathologies, and surprisingly, it maintained its function, even though it was involved in different pathways. miR-625 was reported as downregulated in hepatocellular carcinoma, gastric cancer, and colorectal cancer, and its low expression was associated with local invasion, lymph node, and distant metastasis. Ectopic expression of miR-625 induces suppression of migration and invasion of hepatocellular carcinoma cells by post-transcriptionally inhibiting IGF2BP1. Loss of IGF2BP1 suppressed F-actin polymerization, inhibiting the formation of cell protrusions, required for cell migration. The same effect was observed *in vivo*, where miR-625 overexpression decreased intrahepatic and lung metastasis [103]. Moreover, when it was ectopically induced, miR-625 suppressed the migration and invasion of gastric cancer cells as well as metastasis in nude mice by inhibiting ILK protein synthesis [98]. While the exact signaling pathway was not fully elucidated in colorectal cancer, ectopic miR-625 expression inhibited cell migration and invasion and suppressed colorectal cancer cell metastasis in nude mice [99]. The aforementioned findings highlight miR-625 as an interesting candidate for further *in vivo* studies in order to test its potential for developing a therapeutic microRNA for blocking invasion and metastasis.

A dual and somewhat contradictory behavior can be observed in the case of miR-409. While low miR-409 expression in breast cancer and nonsmall cell lung carcinoma (NSCLC) was associated with poorer prognosis and its ectopic uptake decreased the invasiveness of cancer cells [104, 105], it also seems to exert the negative effect in the case of prostate cancer, where it promotes tumorigenesis and EMT [106, 107]. Qi Song et al. [104] showed that miR-409 inhibits NSCLC cell migration, growth, and proliferation abilities by inhibiting SPIN1 translation. miR-409 downregulates PI3K/AKT pathway in NSCLC and inhibits its downstream targets such as CREB1, BCL2, and Cyclin D. Overexpression of miR-409 led to fewer lung metastases in nude mice, confirming its antimetastatic potential. Interestingly, miR-409 targeted the same pathway and suppressed cell growth and invasion in breast cancer. miR-409-3p inhibits the proliferation, migration, and invasion of breast cancer by targeting and suppressing the AKT expression. miR-409-3p was downregulated in several human tumors compared to their corresponding nontumor tissues [105]. On the other hand, miR-409-entrapped exosomes secreted by cancer-associated fibroblasts (CAFs) and promoted EMT and prostate tumorigenesis. In their study, Josson et al. demonstrated that miR-409-3p was highly expressed in CAFs derived from human patients, and it was correlated with higher Gleason score in prostatic tissues. Moreover, the ectopic expression of miR-409 in normal prostate stromal fibroblasts conferred them a CAF phenotype *in vitro*. Exosome-mediated transport of miR-409 into normal prostate stromal cells induced cell growth and

miRNA	Pathology	Effect	Target	Mechanism	Effect *in vitro* and *in vivo*	Clinical associations	Ref.
miR-148b	Endometrial cancer	Metastasis inhibitor	Inhibits DNMT1	Anti-EMT, increased E-cadherin over vimentin, fibronectin, N-cadherin	Decreased motility and invasion *in vitro*, decreased metastasis *in vivo*	—	[94]
miR-210-3p	Prostate cancer	Metastasis promoter	Inhibits TNIP1 and SOCS1	HIF1-miR-210-3p- > enhances NF-κB signaling inducing EMT	Promoted EMT, invasion, and migration of Pca cells and bone metastasis of Pca cells in mouse	Overexpressed in bone metastatic tissues, correlates with high PSA levels, Gleason grade and bone metastasis status in prostate cancer patients	[95]
miR-210	Breast cancer	Metastasis promoter	Inhibits E-cadherin synthesis	Blocks E-cadherin mRNA by binding to the ORF region	Upregulated in mammosphere cells, induced by hypoxia, promotes invasion, migration, proliferation, and self-renewal, induces EMT by loss of E-cadherin *in vitro* and leads to poorly differentiated tumors, high proliferation, more metastases and higher tumor mass *in vivo*	Upregulated in BCSC CD44+/CD24-sorted from breast cancer tissue samples	[96]
miR-652	Pancreatic cancer	Metastasis inhibitor	Inhibits ZEB1	Acidic microenvironment-miR-652 downregulation-ZEB1 upregulation > EMT	Anti-EMT, reduced migration and invasion, promotes MET *in vitro*, lower tumor mass, fewer metastases, increased expression of E-cadherin vs. vimentin, N-cadherin *in vivo*	Downregulated in pancreatic cancer, correlated with progressive stage, lymphatic invasion, vascular infiltration, distant metastasis	[97]
miR-652	Endometrial cancer	Metastasis promoter	Inhibits RORA	Enhanced b-catenin expression, Wnt-b-catenin signaling pathway	Increased proliferation, and increased metastasis potential *in vitro* and *in vivo*	Upregulated in EC, associated with poor differentiation, poor prognosis, shorter overall survival, and recurrence; not associated with cancer stage, localization, tumor size	[100]

miRNA	Pathology	Effect	Target	Mechanism	Effect *in vitro* and *in vivo*	Clinical associations	Ref.
miR-374a	Breast cancer	Metastasis promoter	Inhibits PTEN, WIF1, WNT5A	Wnt-b-catenin signaling, promoting the transcriptional activity of TCF/LEF	Induces EMT and enhanced motility in MCF7 transfected cells, decreases MDA cells motility in knockout, promotes lung metastases with MCF7 miR-374a transfected cells, impaired MDA-435 metastases by the administration of antagomiR	Upregulated in patients that presented metastases within the 51 months follow up; associated with low WIF1, PTEN, and WNT5A expression in tumor samples; high b-catenin low E-cadherin in miR-374a overexpressing samples	[101]
miR-590-5p	Breast cancer	Metastasis inhibitor	Inhibits PITX2	Blocks Wnt signaling induced by PITX2	Upregulation of miR-590 inhibits EMT genes, inhibits proliferation after 48-72 h, impairs migration and invasion of cancer cells, and promotes smaller tumor size for miR-590 mimic or PITX2 inhibition and less lung and lymphatic metastases in nude mice	Downregulated in breast cancer tissues vs. normal tissue, together with E-cadherin, while PITX2, b-catenin, Wnt-1, N-cadherin, and vimentin are upregulated	[102]
miR-625	Hepatocellular carcinoma	Metastasis inhibitor	Inhibits IGF2BP1	PTEN and Akt signaling downregulation, inhibiting F-actin polymerization	Suppressed migration and invasion, proliferation was not influenced in cell lines, decreased intrahepatic and lung metastasis in mice xenografts	Downregulated in HCC, correlated with aggressiveness of cancer and tumor metastasis	[103]
miR-625	Gastric cancer	Metastasis inhibitor	Inhibits ILK	Suppressed LIMS1-ILK-parvin axis signaling	Reduced migration and invasion rate *in vitro*, suppressed motility and extravasation from vessels, fewer lung metastatic nodes	Downregulated in gastric cancer, associated with lymph-node metastasis; no relation with tumor localization, differentiation, and local invasion	[98]
miR-625	Colorectal cancer	Metastasis inhibitor	—	—	Reduced migration in cancer cell lines; fewer and smaller liver metastases in mouse xenografts	Downregulated in cancer tissues, associated with lymph node and liver metastases and lower overall survival rate in 5 years	[99]

miRNA	Pathology	Effect	Target	Mechanism	Effect *in vitro* and *in vivo*	Clinical associations	Ref.
miR-409	NSCLC	Metastasis inhibitor	Inhibits SPIN1	Downregulation of SPIN1-AKT signaling	Inhibits cell growth, proliferation, and migration *in vitro*; fewer lung metastatic foci *in vivo*	Downregulated in NSLC tissues, correlated with tumor size, stage, pleural invasion, and metastasis; worse overall survival and disease-free survival	[104]
miR-409-3p	Breast cancer	Metastasis inhibitor	Inhibits AKT1 p	Downregulation of PI3K-AKT pathway	Inhibited breast cancer cell proliferation, migration, and invasion suppressed tumor growth *in vivo*	Downregulated to a significant extent in tumor samples, relative to the corresponding nontumor tissues	[105]
miR-409-3p/5p	Prostate cancer	Metastasis promoter	Inhibits RSU1 and STAG2	Upregulation of Ras and Akt signaling	Induces EMT in normal prostate epithelia, promotes tumorigenicity and stemness *in vivo*	Upregulated in human prostatic tissues with higher Gleason score and prostate cancer bone metastasis	[106]
miR-409-3p/5p	Prostate cancer	Metastasis promoter	Inhibits STAG2 and RSU1	Upregulation of Ras-ILK signaling	Induction of an EMT phenotype, decreased E-cadherin, increased vimentin, b-actin and downregulation of tumor suppressing genes	Higher miR-409 expression in the stromal fibroblasts, correlated with higher Gleason score in prostatic tissues	[107]
miR-409-5p	Breast cancer	Metastasis promoter	Inhibits RSU1	Upregulation of Ras signaling	Induces proliferation and migration in cancer cells and tumor growth in mice xenografts	Upregulation in breast can carcinoma tissues, correlated with shorter survival	[108]

Table 2.
In vitro and in vivo validated miRNAs related to EMT, invasion, and metastasis that could represent future therapy targets.

EMT *in vitro* and *in vivo.* In this case, the predicted targets of miR-409 were the tumor-suppressor proteins STAG2 and RSU1, which appeared downregulated [108]. Considering these, it would be worth exploring if miR-409 has a positive or a negative impact over EMT and metastasis in more human cancers, and if it could be taken into consideration as a future miRNA therapy target.

Table 2 comprises a set of microRNAs that were evaluated both *in vitro* and *in vivo*, while also being analyzed in tumor samples, in correlation with the clinical outcome of the patients. As it can be easily observed, the effect of microRNAs in modulating EMT and metastasis-related pathways varies in different cancer types. In certain situations, the same microRNA can induce completely opposite outcomes by targeting multiple signaling pathways. This would be one of the biggest challenges that need to be overcome when designing new microRNA-based therapeutic compounds, and it is, at the same time, an interesting research niche worth exploring, especially for miR-625, that maintained its anti-EMT function in three different cancer types (hepatocellular carcinoma, gastric cancer, and colorectal cancer) and miR-409 that is able to target multiple pathways with opposing effects in NSCLC, breast cancer, and prostate cancer.

7. Conclusions

miRNAs represent key modulators of the human genome because of their capacity to affect up to 60% of protein-coding genes. In cancer, genetic and epigenetic events lead to the alteration of miRNA expression and consequently their mRNA target genes. Functional studies have demonstrated that miRNA modulation in tumor cells causes changes in the phenotype, leading to increased apoptosis and cell death, suppression of tumor development, invasion, and metastasis by inhibiting the oncogenic miRNAs (oncomiRs) and/or substituting the deficient tumor suppressive miRNAs (TS-miRNAs). Considering the encouraging preclinical and clinical data, miRNA-based therapy could become a reliable tool in cancer management.

Acknowledgements

The work for this chapter was supported by the UEFISCDI Program-PN-III-P2-2.1-PED-2016-1750.

Conflict of interest

The authors declare no conflict of interest.

Author details

Ovidiu Balacescu[1,2*], Simona Visan[1], Oana Baldasici[1,3], Loredana Balacescu[1,2], Catalin Vlad[4,5] and Patriciu Achimas-Cadariu[4,5]

1 Department of Functional Genomics, Proteomics and Experimental Pathology, The Oncology Institute "Prof. Dr. Ion Chiricuta", Cluj-Napoca, Romania

2 Department of Medical Oncology, University of Medicine and Pharmacy "Iuliu Hatieganu", Cluj-Napoca, Romania

3 Faculty of Pharmacy, University of Medicine and Pharmacy "Iuliu Hatieganu", Cluj-Napoca, Romania

4 Department of Surgical and Gynecological Oncology, University of Medicine and Pharmacy "Iuliu Hatieganu", Cluj-Napoca, Romania

5 Department of Surgery, The Oncology Institute "Prof. Dr. Ion Chiricuta", Cluj-Napoca, Romania

*Address all correspondence to: obalacescu@yahoo.com

IntechOpen

© 2018 The Author(s). Licensee IntechOpen. This chapter is distributed under the terms of the Creative Commons Attribution License (http://creativecommons.org/licenses/by/3.0), which permits unrestricted use, distribution, and reproduction in any medium, provided the original work is properly cited. CC BY

References

[1] Society AC. Global Cancer Facts & Figures. 3rd ed. Atlanta: American Cancer Society; 2015

[2] Ferlay J, Soerjomataram I, Dikshit R, Eser S, Mathers C, Rebelo M, et al. Cancer incidence and mortality worldwide: Sources, methods and major patterns in GLOBOCAN 2012. International Journal of Cancer. 2015;**136**(5):E359-E386

[3] Chaffer CL, Weinberg RA. A perspective on cancer cell metastasis. Science. 2011;**331**(6024):1559-1564

[4] Hanahan D, Weinberg RA. Hallmarks of cancer: The next generation. Cell. 2011;**144**(5):646-674

[5] Polyak K, Weinberg RA. Transitions between epithelial and mesenchymal states: Acquisition of malignant and stem cell traits. Nature Reviews. Cancer. 2009;**9**(4):265-273

[6] Jolly MK, Tripathi SC, Somarelli JA, Hanash SM, Levine H. Epithelial/mesenchymal plasticity: How have quantitative mathematical models helped improve our understanding? Molecular Oncology. 2017;**11**(7):739-754

[7] Pennisi E. Genomics. ENCODE project writes eulogy for junk DNA. Science 2012;**337**(6099):1159-1161

[8] Ambros V. The evolution of our thinking about microRNAs. Nature Medicine. 2008;**14**(10):1036-1040

[9] Kim VN, Han J, Siomi MC. Biogenesis of small RNAs in animals. Nature Reviews. Molecular Cell Biology. 2009;**10**(2):126-139

[10] Lewis BP, Burge CB, Bartel DP. Conserved seed pairing, often flanked by adenosines, indicates that thousands of human genes are microRNA targets. Cell. 2005;**120**(1):15-20

[11] Krek A, Grun D, Poy MN, Wolf R, Rosenberg L, Epstein EJ, et al. Combinatorial microRNA target predictions. Nature Genetics. 2005;**37**(5):495-500

[12] Coronnello C, Benos PV. ComiR: Combinatorial microRNA target prediction tool. Nucleic Acids Research. 2013;**41**(Web Server issue):W159-W164

[13] Friedman Y, Karsenty S, Linial M. miRror-suite: Decoding coordinated regulation by microRNAs. Database (Oxford). 6 Jun 2014;**2014**:pii:bau043. DOI: 10.1093/database/bau043

[14] Kozomara A, Griffiths-Jones S. miRBase: Annotating high confidence microRNAs using deep sequencing data. Nucleic Acids Research. 2014;**42**(Database issue):D68-D73

[15] Calin GA, Dumitru CD, Shimizu M, Bichi R, Zupo S, Noch E, et al. Frequent deletions and down-regulation of micro-RNA genes miR15 and miR16 at 13q14 in chronic lymphocytic leukemia. Proceedings of the National Academy of Sciences of the United States of America. 2002;**99**(24):15524-15529

[16] Cimmino A, Calin GA, Fabbri M, Iorio MV, Ferracin M, Shimizu M, et al. miR-15 and miR-16 induce apoptosis by targeting BCL2. Proceedings of the National Academy of Sciences of the United States of America. 2005;**102**(39):13944-13949

[17] Calin GA, Liu CG, Sevignani C, Ferracin M, Felli N, Dumitru CD, et al. MicroRNA profiling reveals distinct signatures in B cell chronic lymphocytic leukemias. Proceedings of the National Academy of Sciences of the United States of America. 2004;**101**(32):11755-11760

[18] Lu J, Getz G, Miska EA, Alvarez-Saavedra E, Lamb J, Peck D, et al.

MicroRNA expression profiles classify human cancers. Nature. 2005;**435**(7043):834-838

[19] Weber JA, Baxter DH, Zhang S, Huang DY, Huang KH, Lee MJ, et al. The microRNA spectrum in 12 body fluids. Clinical Chemistry. 2010;**56**(11):1733-1741

[20] Lan H, Lu H, Wang X, Jin H. MicroRNAs as potential biomarkers in cancer: Opportunities and challenges. BioMed Research International. 2015;**2015**:125094

[21] Hata A, Kashima R. Dysregulation of microRNA biogenesis machinery in cancer. Critical Reviews in Biochemistry and Molecular Biology. 2016;**51**(3):121-134

[22] Di Leva G, Garofalo M, Croce CM. MicroRNAs in cancer. Annual Review of Pathology. 2014;**9**:287-314

[23] Croce CM. Causes and consequences of microRNA dysregulation in cancer. Nature Reviews. Genetics. 2009;**10**(10):704-714

[24] Zhang B, Pan X, Cobb GP, Anderson TA. microRNAs as oncogenes and tumor suppressors. Developmental Biology. 2007;**302**(1):1-12

[25] Romero-Cordoba SL, Salido-Guadarrama I, Rodriguez-Dorantes M, Hidalgo-Miranda A. miRNA biogenesis: Biological impact in the development of cancer. Cancer Biology & Therapy. 2014;**15**(11):1444-1455

[26] Berindan-Neagoe I, Monroig Pdel C, Pasculli B, Calin GA. MicroRNAome genome: A treasure for cancer diagnosis and therapy. CA: A Cancer Journal for Clinicians. 2014;**64**(5):311-336

[27] Shah MY, Ferrajoli A, Sood AK, Lopez-Berestein G, Calin GA. microRNA therapeutics in cancer—An emerging concept. eBioMedicine. 2016;**12**:34-42

[28] Garzon R, Marcucci G, Croce CM. Targeting microRNAs in cancer: Rationale, strategies and challenges. Nature Reviews. Drug Discovery. 2010;**9**(10):775-789

[29] Vester B, Wengel J. LNA (locked nucleic acid): High-affinity targeting of complementary RNA and DNA. Biochemistry. 2004;**43**(42):13233-13241

[30] Elmen J, Lindow M, Schutz S, Lawrence M, Petri A, Obad S, et al. LNA-mediated microRNA silencing in non-human primates. Nature. 2008;**452**(7189):896-899

[31] Krützfeldt J, Rajewsky N, Braich R, Rajeev KG, Tuschl T, Manoharan M, et al. Silencing of microRNAs in vivo with 'antagomirs'. Nature. 2005;**438**(7068):685-689

[32] Ebert MS, Neilson JR, Sharp PA. MicroRNA sponges: Competitive inhibitors of small RNAs in mammalian cells. Nature Methods. 2007;**4**(9):721-726

[33] Monroig Pdel C, Chen L, Zhang S, Calin GA. Small molecule compounds targeting miRNAs for cancer therapy. Advanced Drug Delivery Reviews. 2015;**81**:104-116

[34] Griveau A, Bejaud J, Anthiya S, Avril S, Autret D, Garcion E. Silencing of miR-21 by locked nucleic acid-lipid nanocapsule complexes sensitize human glioblastoma cells to radiation-induced cell death. International Journal of Pharmaceutics. 2013;**454**(2):765-774

[35] Bader AG, Brown D, Winkler M. The promise of microRNA replacement therapy. Cancer Research. 2010;**70**(18):7027-7030

[36] Kota J, Chivukula RR, O'Donnell KA, Wentzel EA, Montgomery CL, Hwang HW, et al. Therapeutic microRNA delivery

suppresses tumorigenesis in a murine liver cancer model. Cell. 2009;**137**(6):1005-1017

[37] Zhang J, Li S, Li L, Li M, Guo C, Yao J, et al. Exosome and exosomal microRNA: Trafficking, sorting, and function. Genomics, Proteomics & Bioinformatics. 2015;**13**(1):17-24

[38] Fabbri M, Paone A, Calore F, Galli R, Gaudio E, Santhanam R, et al. MicroRNAs bind to toll-like receptors to induce prometastatic inflammatory response. Proceedings of the National Academy of Sciences of the United States of America. 2012;**109**(31):E2110-E2116

[39] Aagaard L, Rossi JJ. RNAi therapeutics: Principles, prospects and challenges. Advanced Drug Delivery Reviews. 2007;**59**(2-3):75-86

[40] Bakhshandeh B, Soleimani M, Hafizi M, Ghaemi N. A comparative study on nonviral genetic modifications in cord blood and bone marrow mesenchymal stem cells. Cytotechnology. 2012;**64**(5):523-540

[41] Hosseinahli N, Aghapour M, Duijf PHG, Baradaran B. Treating cancer with microRNA replacement therapy: A literature review. Journal of Cellular Physiology. 2018;**233**(8):5574-5588

[42] Ibrahim AF, Weirauch U, Thomas M, Grunweller A, Hartmann RK, Aigner A. MicroRNA replacement therapy for miR-145 and miR-33a is efficacious in a model of colon carcinoma. Cancer Research. 2011;**71**(15):5214-5224

[43] Kaban K, Salva E, Akbuga J. The effects of chitosan/miR-200c nanoplexes on different stages of cancers in breast cancer cell lines. European Journal of Pharmaceutical Sciences. 2016;**95**:103-110

[44] Kaban K, Salva E, Akbuga J. In vitro dose studies on chitosan nanoplexes for microRNA delivery in breast cancer cells. Nucleic Acid Therapeutics. 2017;**27**(1):45-55

[45] Hao Z, Fan W, Hao J, Wu X, Zeng GQ, Zhang LJ, et al. Efficient delivery of micro RNA to bone-metastatic prostate tumors by using aptamer-conjugated atelocollagen in vitro and in vivo. Drug Delivery. 2016;**23**(3):874-881

[46] Trang P, Medina PP, Wiggins JF, Ruffino L, Kelnar K, Omotola M, et al. Regression of murine lung tumors by the let-7 microRNA. Oncogene. 2010;**29**(11):1580-1587

[47] Trang P, Wiggins JF, Daige CL, Cho C, Omotola M, Brown D, et al. Systemic delivery of tumor suppressor microRNA mimics using a neutral lipid emulsion inhibits lung tumors in mice. Molecular Therapy. 2011;**19**(6):1116-1122

[48] Dalmay T, Edwards DR. MicroRNAs and the hallmarks of cancer. Oncogene. 2006;**25**(46):6170-6175

[49] Nicoloso MS, Spizzo R, Shimizu M, Rossi S, Calin GA. MicroRNAs—The micro steering wheel of tumour metastases. Nature Reviews. Cancer. 2009;**9**(4):293-302

[50] Valeri N, Gasparini P, Fabbri M, Braconi C, Veronese A, Lovat F, et al. Modulation of mismatch repair and genomic stability by miR-155. Proceedings of the National Academy of Sciences of the United States of America. 2010;**107**(15):6982-6987

[51] Guessous F, Alvarado-Velez M, Marcinkiewicz L, Zhang Y, Kim J, Heister S, et al. Oncogenic effects of miR-10b in glioblastoma stem cells. Journal of Neuro-Oncology. 2013;**112**(2):153-163

[52] Ma L, Reinhardt F, Pan E, Soutschek J, Bhat B, Marcusson EG, et al. Therapeutic silencing of miR-10b inhibits metastasis in a mouse mammary tumor model. Nature Biotechnology. 2010;**28**(4):341-347

[53] Callegari E, Elamin BK, Giannone F, Milazzo M, Altavilla G, Fornari F, et al. Liver tumorigenicity promoted by microRNA-221 in a mouse transgenic model. Hepatology. 2012;**56**(3):1025-1033

[54] Qin J, Luo M. MicroRNA-221 promotes colorectal cancer cell invasion and metastasis by targeting RECK. FEBS Letters. 2014;**588**(1):99-104

[55] Brognara E, Fabbri E, Aimi F, Manicardi A, Bianchi N, Finotti A, et al. Peptide nucleic acids targeting miR-221 modulate p27Kip1 expression in breast cancer MDA-MB-231 cells. International Journal of Oncology. 2012;**41**(6):2119-2127

[56] Gallo Cantafio ME, Nielsen BS, Mignogna C, Arbitrio M, Botta C, Frandsen NM, Rolfo C, Tagliaferri P, Tassone P, Di Martino MT. Pharmacokinetics and pharmacodynamics of a 13-mer LNA-inhibitor-miR-221 in mice and non-human primates. Molecular Therapy Nucleic Acids. 21 Jun 2016;**5**(6). DOI: 10.1038/mtna.2016.36

[57] Chang TC, Wentzel EA, Kent OA, Ramachandran K, Mullendore M, Lee KH, et al. Transactivation of miR-34a by p53 broadly influences gene expression and promotes apoptosis. Molecular Cell. 2007;**26**(5):745-752

[58] Chang TC, Yu D, Lee YS, Wentzel EA, Arking DE, West KM, et al. Widespread microRNA repression by Myc contributes to tumorigenesis. Nature Genetics. 2008;**40**(1):43-50

[59] Lodygin D, Tarasov V, Epanchintsev A, Berking C, Knyazeva T, Korner H, et al. Inactivation of miR-34a by aberrant CpG methylation in multiple types of cancer. Cell Cycle. 2008;**7**(16):2591-2600

[60] He L, He X, Lim LP, de Stanchina E, Xuan Z, Liang Y, et al. A microRNA component of the p53 tumour suppressor network. Nature. 2007;**447**(7148):1130-1134

[61] Gallardo E, Navarro A, Vinolas N, Marrades RM, Diaz T, Gel B, et al. miR-34a as a prognostic marker of relapse in surgically resected non-small-cell lung cancer. Carcinogenesis. 2009;**30**(11):1903-1909

[62] O'Day E, Lal A. MicroRNAs and their target gene networks in breast cancer. Breast Cancer Research. 2010;**12**(2):201

[63] Corney DC, Hwang CI, Matoso A, Vogt M, Flesken-Nikitin A, Godwin AK, et al. Frequent downregulation of miR-34 family in human ovarian cancers. Clinical Cancer Research. 2010;**16**(4):1119-1128

[64] Girardi C, De Pitta C, Casara S, Sales G, Lanfranchi G, Celotti L, et al. Analysis of miRNA and mRNA expression profiles highlights alterations in ionizing radiation response of human lymphocytes under modeled microgravity. PLoS One. 2012;**7**(2):e31293

[65] Josson S, Sung SY, Lao K, Chung LW, Johnstone PA. Radiation modulation of microRNA in prostate cancer cell lines. The Prostate. 2008;**68**(15):1599-1606

[66] Nikiforova MN, Gandhi M, Kelly L, Nikiforov YE. MicroRNA dysregulation in human thyroid cells following exposure to ionizing radiation. Thyroid. 2011;**21**(3):261-266

[67] Daige CL, Wiggins JF, Priddy L, Nelligan-Davis T, Zhao J, Brown D. Systemic delivery of a miR34a mimic

as a potential therapeutic for liver cancer. Molecular Cancer Therapeutics. 2014;**13**(10):2352-2360

[68] Bader AG. miR-34—A microRNA replacement therapy is headed to the clinic. Frontiers in Genetics. 2012;**3**:120

[69] Bandi N, Zbinden S, Gugger M, Arnold M, Kocher V, Hasan L, et al. miR-15a and miR-16 are implicated in cell cycle regulation in a Rb-dependent manner and are frequently deleted or down-regulated in non-small cell lung cancer. Cancer Research. 2009;**69**(13):5553-5559

[70] Bonci D, Coppola V, Musumeci M, Addario A, Giuffrida R, Memeo L, et al. The miR-15a-miR-16-1 cluster controls prostate cancer by targeting multiple oncogenic activities. Nature Medicine. 2008;**14**(11):1271-1277

[71] Reid G, Pel ME, Kirschner MB, Cheng YY, Mugridge N, Weiss J, et al. Restoring expression of miR-16: A novel approach to therapy for malignant pleural mesothelioma. Annals of Oncology. 2013;**24**(12):3128-3135

[72] Takeshita F, Patrawala L, Osaki M, Takahashi RU, Yamamoto Y, Kosaka N, et al. Systemic delivery of synthetic microRNA-16 inhibits the growth of metastatic prostate tumors via downregulation of multiple cell-cycle genes. Molecular Therapy. 2010;**18**(1):181-187

[73] Kluiver J, Poppema S, de Jong D, Blokzijl T, Harms G, Jacobs S, et al. BIC and miR-155 are highly expressed in Hodgkin, primary mediastinal and diffuse large B cell lymphomas. The Journal of Pathology. 2005;**207**(2):243-249

[74] Calin GA, Ferracin M, Cimmino A, Di Leva G, Shimizu M, Wojcik SE, et al. A MicroRNA signature associated with prognosis and progression in chronic lymphocytic leukemia. The New England Journal of Medicine. 2005;**353**(17):1793-1801

[75] Yanaihara N, Caplen N, Bowman E, Seike M, Kumamoto K, Yi M, et al. Unique microRNA molecular profiles in lung cancer diagnosis and prognosis. Cancer Cell. 2006;**9**(3):189-198

[76] Iorio MV, Ferracin M, Liu CG, Veronese A, Spizzo R, Sabbioni S, et al. MicroRNA gene expression deregulation in human breast cancer. Cancer Research. 2005;**65**(16):7065-7070

[77] Garzon R, Volinia S, Liu CG, Fernandez-Cymering C, Palumbo T, Pichiorri F, et al. MicroRNA signatures associated with cytogenetics and prognosis in acute myeloid leukemia. Blood. 2008;**111**(6):3183-3189

[78] Volinia S, Calin GA, Liu CG, Ambs S, Cimmino A, Petrocca F, et al. A microRNA expression signature of human solid tumors defines cancer gene targets. Proceedings of the National Academy of Sciences of the United States of America. 2006;**103**(7):2257-2261

[79] Philippidou D, Schmitt M, Moser D, Margue C, Nazarov PV, Muller A, et al. Signatures of microRNAs and selected microRNA target genes in human melanoma. Cancer Research. 2010;**70**(10):4163-4173

[80] Gasparini P, Lovat F, Fassan M, Casadei L, Cascione L, Jacob NK, et al. Protective role of miR-155 in breast cancer through RAD51 targeting impairs homologous recombination after irradiation. Proceedings of the National Academy of Sciences of the United States of America. 2014;**111**(12):4536-4541

[81] Pouliot LM, Chen YC, Bai J, Guha R, Martin SE, Gottesman MM, et al.

Cisplatin sensitivity mediated by WEE1 and CHK1 is mediated by miR-155 and the miR-15 family. Cancer Research. 2012;**72**(22):5945-5955

[82] Hoshino A, Costa-Silva B, Shen TL, Rodrigues G, Hashimoto A, Tesic Mark M, et al. Tumour exosome integrins determine organotropic metastasis. Nature. 2015;**527**(7578):329-335

[83] David S, Hong Y-KK, Brenner AJ, Sachdev JC, Ejadi S, Borad MJ, et al. MRX34, a liposomal miR-34 mimic, in patients with advanced solid tumors: Final dose-escalation results from a first-in-human phase I trial of microRNA therapy. Journal of Clinical Oncology. 2016;**34**(15_suppl):2508

[84] Cortez MA, Ivan C, Valdecanas D, Wang X, Peltier HJ, Ye Y, et al. PDL1 regulation by p53 via miR-34. Journal of the National Cancer Institute. 17 Nov 2015;**108**(1):pii:djv303. DOI: 10.1093/jnci/djv303

[85] Reid GW M, Kirschner MB, Mugridge N, Weiss J, Brahmbhatt H, et al. Targeted delivery of a synthetic microRNA-based mimic as an approach to cancer therapy. Cancer Research. AACR; 2015;**75**(15 Suppl):Abstract nr 3976. DOI: 10.1158/1538-7445.AM2015-3976

[86] Van Zandwijk N, Pavlakis N, Kao S, Clarke S, Lee A, Brahmbhatt H, et al. MesomiR 1: A phase I study of TargomiRs in patients with refractory malignant pleural mesothelioma (MPM) and lung cancer (NSCLC). Annals of Oncology 2015;**26**(suppl_2):ii16

[87] Christopher AF, Kaur RP, Kaur G, Kaur A, Gupta V, Bansal P. MicroRNA therapeutics: Discovering novel targets and developing specific therapy. Perspectives in Clinical Research. 2016;**7**(2):68-74

[88] Rupaimoole R, Slack FJ. MicroRNA therapeutics: Towards a new era for the management of cancer and other diseases. Nature Reviews. Drug Discovery. 2017;**16**(3):203-222

[89] Rupaimoole R, Calin GA, Lopez-Berestein G, Sood AK. miRNA deregulation in cancer cells and the tumor microenvironment. Cancer Discovery. 2016;**6**(3):235-246

[90] Peinado H, Zhang H, Matei IR, Costa-Silva B, Hoshino A, Rodrigues G, et al. Pre-metastatic niches: Organ-specific homes for metastases. Nature Reviews. Cancer. 2017;**17**(5):302-317

[91] Lamouille S, Xu J, Derynck R. Molecular mechanisms of epithelial-mesenchymal transition. Nature Reviews. Molecular Cell Biology. 2014;**15**(3):178-196

[92] Vuoriluoto K, Haugen H, Kiviluoto S, Mpindi JP, Nevo J, Gjerdrum C, et al. Vimentin regulates EMT induction by Slug and oncogenic H-Ras and migration by governing Axl expression in breast cancer. Oncogene. 2011;**30**(12):1436-1448

[93] Zheng H, Kang Y. Multilayer control of the EMT master regulators. Oncogene. 2014;**33**(14):1755-1763

[94] Li BL, Lu W, Qu JJ, Ye L, Du GQ, Wan XP. Loss of exosomal miR-148b from cancer-associated fibroblasts promotes endometrial cancer cell invasion and cancer metastasis. Journal of Cellular Physiology. 26 Aug 2018. DOI: 10.1002/jcp.27111. [Epub ahead of print]

[95] Ren D, Yang Q, Dai Y, Guo W, Du H, Song L, et al. Oncogenic miR-210-3p promotes prostate cancer cell EMT and bone metastasis via NF-kappaB signaling pathway. Molecular Cancer. 2017;**16**(1):117

[96] Tang T, Yang Z, Zhu Q, Wu Y, Sun K, Alahdal M, et al. Up-regulation of miR-210 induced by a hypoxic microenvironment promotes breast cancer stem cells metastasis, proliferation, and self-renewal by targeting E-cadherin. FASEB Journal. 6 Sep 2018:fj201801013R. DOI: 10.1096/fj.201801013R. [Epub ahead of print]

[97] Deng S, Li X, Niu Y, Zhu S, Jin Y, Deng S, et al. MiR-652 inhibits acidic microenvironment-induced epithelial-mesenchymal transition of pancreatic cancer cells by targeting ZEB1. Oncotarget. 2015;**6**(37):39661-39675

[98] Wang M, Li C, Nie H, Lv X, Qu Y, Yu B, et al. Down-regulated miR-625 suppresses invasion and metastasis of gastric cancer by targeting ILK. FEBS Letters. 2012;**586**(16):2382-2238

[99] Lou X, Qi X, Zhang Y, Long H, Yang J. Decreased expression of microRNA-625 is associated with tumor metastasis and poor prognosis in patients with colorectal cancer. Journal of Surgical Oncology. 2013;**108**(4):230-235

[100] Sun X, Dongol S, Qiu C, Xu Y, Sun C, Zhang Z, et al. miR-652 promotes tumor proliferation and metastasis by targeting RORA in endometrial cancer. Molecular Cancer Research. 9 Aug 2018. DOI: 10.1158/1541-7786.MCR-18-0267. [Epub ahead of print]

[101] Cai J, Guan H, Fang L, Yang Y, Zhu X, Yuan J, et al. MicroRNA-374a activates Wnt/beta-catenin signaling to promote breast cancer metastasis. The Journal of Clinical Investigation. 2013;**123**(2):566-579

[102] Gao J, Yu SR, Yuan Y, Zhang LL, Lu JW, Feng JF, Hu SN. MicroRNA-590-5p functions as a tumor suppressor in breast cancer conferring inhibitory effects on cell migration, invasion, and epithelial-mesenchymal transition by downregulating the Wnt-β-catenin signaling pathway. Journal of Cellular Physiology. 7 Sep 2018. DOI: 10.1002/jcp.27056. [Epub ahead of print]

[103] Zhou X, Zhang CZ, Lu SX, Chen GG, Li LZ, Liu LL, et al. miR-625 suppresses tumour migration and invasion by targeting IGF2BP1 in hepatocellular carcinoma. Oncogene. 2015;**34**(8):965-977

[104] Song Q, Ji Q, Xiao J, Li F, Wang L, Chen Y, Xu Y, Jiao S. miR-409 inhibits human non-small-cell lung cancer progression by directly targeting SPIN1. Molecular Therapy Nucleic Acids. 1 Sep 2018;**13**:154-163. DOI: 10.1016/j.omtn.2018.08.020. [Epub ahead of print]

[105] Zhang G, Liu Z, Xu H, Yang Q. miR-409-3p suppresses breast cancer cell growth and invasion by targeting Akt1. Biochemical and Biophysical Research Communications. 2016;**469**(2):189-195

[106] Josson S, Gururajan M, Hu P, Shao C, Chu GY, Zhau HE, et al. miR-409-3p/−5p promotes tumorigenesis, epithelial-to-mesenchymal transition, and bone metastasis of human prostate cancer. Clinical Cancer Research. 2014;**20**(17):4636-4646

[107] Josson S, Gururajan M, Sung SY, Hu P, Shao C, Zhau HE, et al. Stromal fibroblast-derived miR-409 promotes epithelial-to-mesenchymal transition and prostate tumorigenesis. Oncogene. 2015;**34**(21):2690-2699

[108] Yu H, Xing H, Han W, Wang Y, Qi T, Song C, et al. MicroRNA-409-5p is upregulated in breast cancer and its downregulation inhibits cancer development through downstream target of RSU1. Tumour Biology. 2017;**39**(5):1010428317701647

Chapter 4

Oncoproteins Targeting: Antibodies, Antisense, Triple-helix. Case of Anti IGF-I Cancer Immunogene Therapy

Jerzy Trojan

Abstract

AFP and IGF-I oncoproteins were introduced as biomarkers for cancer diagnosis and targeted in cancer therapy on protein level, but also on transcription and translation levels. The protein level was targeted using an injection of antibodies or radiolabeled proteins. The transcription and translation levels were targeted by triple helix and antisense technologies, respectively. AFP was especially useful for diagnosis and therapy of liver cancer, IGF-I was applied in diagnosis and therapy of colon, prostate, liver, uterus, ovary and brain tumors. The most spectacular results were obtained with IGF-I anti-gene strategy. IGF-I antisense (AS)/triple helix (TH) gene therapy was successfully introduced in clinical trial in the USA and Europe. When using IGF-I anti-gene therapy, cancer cells provided from biopsies were transfected *in vitro* with IGF-I AS, IGF-I TH expression vectors. A decrease in IGF-I gene expression of 80 and 60% was demonstrated when using TH and AS technologies, respectively. These transfected cells expressing MHC-I molecules, while injected *in vivo*, induced immune antitumor response mediated by CD8 lymphocytes. The median survival of treated glioblastoma patients was 21–22 months. IGF-I AS/TH immunogene therapy constitutes one of the most promising approaches in cancer therapy, and more specifically when it comes to glioblastoma treatment.

Keywords: cancer, glioma, alpha-fetoprotein, IGF-I, diagnostic, antibodies, antisense, triple helix, immunotherapy

1. Introduction

Oncoproteins like alpha-fetoprotein (AFP), serum albumin (AS), and growth factors such as GH, IGF, TGF-beta, and EGF are present in embryo-fetal tissues and reappear in neoplastic developing tissues, including the central nervous system; this concerns especially AFP [1–8] and IGF-I [9–17]. AFP is present in both neural and glial developing and cancerous cells, whereas IGF-I is only present in glial developing and tumoral cells [10, 18]. This striking difference has helped us orientate a strategy to manage the most malignant brain tumor expressing IGF-I gene—glioblastoma.

IGF-I plays an important role in growth as a mediator of growth hormone [19–21]. Blocking IGF-I synthesis induces apoptotic and immunogenic phenomena [12, 22]. Both phenomena, apoptosis and immunogenicity, related to arrest of IGF-I expression

IntechOpen

in neoplastic glial cells, were used to prepare antitumor cell vaccines for therapy of brain malignant tumor—glioblastoma [12, 23].

An efficient strategy targeting IGF-I was established by construction of vectors stopping the synthesis of this oncoprotein on translation and transcription levels: vectors expressing either IGF-I antisense RNA or IGF-I RNA forming RNA-DNA triple helix, respectively. The glioma cells transfected with these vectors, when injected *in vivo* in animals bearing tumors like glioma or teratocarcinoma or applied in clinical treatment of glioblastoma patients, induced an immune antitumor effect (CD8+) accompanied by increase of the median survival of patients (successful clinical results obtained in the USA, E.U., China) [22, 23].

2. Oncoproteins in diagnostic: AFP and IGF-I

2.1 AFP

AFP is present in normal and neoplastic developing tissues [1, 24–26]. The presence of AFP seems to be related to the stage of cell and tissue differentiation. AFP is absent from either undifferentiated or fully differentiated cells [24].

The localization of AFP was compared with that of another oncoprotein—serum albumin, SA. SA-mRNA gave a strong signal in differentiating structures as well as in undifferentiated cell clusters. AFP-mRNA was observed only in differentiating structures; this observation was especially useful in the clinical diagnostic of hepatocarcinoma [4, 27].

During an experiment with teratocarcinoma-bearing mice injected intraperitoneally with J-125 radiolabeled SA and AFP, significant accumulations of both SA and AFP were demonstrated in the tumors, SA being about 3-fold higher than that of AFP after normalization to quantity of uptake in liver. In the case of comparatively studied neuroblastoma presenting only neuroblastic components (different from teratocarcinoma containing both neuroectoblastic and neuroblastic elements), the accumulation of radiolabeled SA and AFP showed relationship 1:1. External *in vivo* photo scanning confirmed this relationship of accumulated radiolabeled proteins in both studied tumors; the last observations were useful for differential diagnosis of tumors [4, 27–36].

AFP may be used to advantage in radio tracing experiments, since this isologous protein is not expected to induce hypersensitivity reactions. On the other hand, and contrary to SA, the extremely low serum levels of AFP in adult individuals should minimize effects due to competition with endogenous protein. This makes AFP a good candidate for tumor biomarker by imaging techniques. The diagnosis and therapies of CNS tumors including neuroblastoma are always a subject of discussion [36–39].

2.2 IGF-I

Another oncodevelopmental antigen, an insulin like-growth factor, IGF-I [20, 40–43], is present in glioma cells but absent in neuroblastoma cells [18]; neuroblastic cells express IGF-II [27]. These observations permitted to study separately, using IGF-I and IGF-II as the oncoprotein markers, glial and neural tumors [13, 15, 20, 40–42, 44–46].

Comparative studies of AFP, IGF-I, IGF-II presence in neoplastic cells [3, 4, 18] have demonstrated that IGF-I constitutes an essential target for genetic testing. IGF-I, similarly to AFP, is involved in tissue development and differentiation, especially in the development of the nervous system [9, 15, 19, 20, 47–51]. According to

Baserga [43], IGF-I is one of the most important growth factors related to normal and neoplastic differentiation [50, 52–54].

The elements of IGF-I related transduction pathway (IRS/PI3K-PKC/PDK1/AKT-Bcl2/GSK3/GS) [55, 56] were also considered as targets for diagnostic [9, 55, 57–66]. The relationship between IGF-I and IGF binding proteins are being introduced in clinical diagnostics as one of the indicators of precancerous development [67].

IGF-I becomes useful in molecular diagnostic of neonatal CNS malformations and tumors [5, 9, 13, 39, 68, 69]. Diagnosis and treatment should logically be related, at first using IGF-I gene testing for diagnosis [13, 21, 70], and then targeting IGF-I gene through special therapy, such as cancer gene therapy, especially therapy of gliomas [11, 22, 71–73].

3. IGF-I and anti-gene immunotherapy

3.1 Protein, translation and transcription levels

To target an oncoprotein directly on protein level, the strategy of antibodies was explored. Cancers treated by use of antibodies was in general not efficient.

The treatment of any cancer, especially hepatocarcinoma, demands a permanent perfusion, *per vena porta*, of anti AFP antibodies. The arrest of perfusion has produced the reappearance of cancer. Similar observation has been made when using antibodies against growth factors.

The only possibility was to stop the synthesis of the oncoprotein on the translation or on the transcription level of the concerned gene, and directly in the cancer cells. This hypothesis and our knowledge of chemistry was an epistemological problem, pointed out by Mosquera "how to integrate the knowledge of chemistry with technique" [74].

As to glioma malignant tumor, glioblastoma (the mortality remains close to 100%), new or proposed therapies are based generally either on immune treatment or on immuno-gene strategies [75, 76]. In order to define new therapies, the different techniques for inhibitors [9], and the anti-gene strategy (either antisense, AS, or triple helix, TH, approaches) were investigated [61] (**Figure 1**).

The AS technology [77, 78] has permitted us to establish new and successful gene therapy strategies targeting glioma's growth factors [11, 79] and have now been introduced into clinical trials. Other recently introduced technologies include those of triple helix, TH [80–83], as well as potentially useful siRNA [84, 85] and miRNA (microRNA) [82, 83, 86, 87]. The role of 21–23 mer double-stranded RNA (siRNA) in the silencing of genes is strongly similar to that of the TH DNA mechanism, which also involves 23 mer RNA [81]. Whether or not siRNA technology or miRNA knockdown will supplant the AS and TH oligodeoxynucleotide approaches remains in question at this time [83, 85, 87–90]. AS methodology is currently being standardized to be largely used in clinical trials [18, 89].

As to TH strategy, the oligonucleotides are targeted to double stranded DNA containing polypurine-polypyrimidine sequences that readily form triple helixes. The studies of triple helix strategy have shown that an RNA strand containing a 23-nucleotide (nt) oligopurine sequence [80, 86, 87] may be capable of forming triple helix structures with an oligopurine-oligopyrimidine sequence of the IGF-I gene as well in cultured rat C6 glioma as in rat CNS-1 glioma, and in mouse PCC-4 cells [86]. Although we cannot exclude other mechanisms, triple helix formation remains the most plausible possibility for the inhibition of IGF-I gene expression [86]. The arrest of IGF-I synthesis suggests that the RNA strand, which forms the triple helix, has inhibited gene transcription in glioma cells.

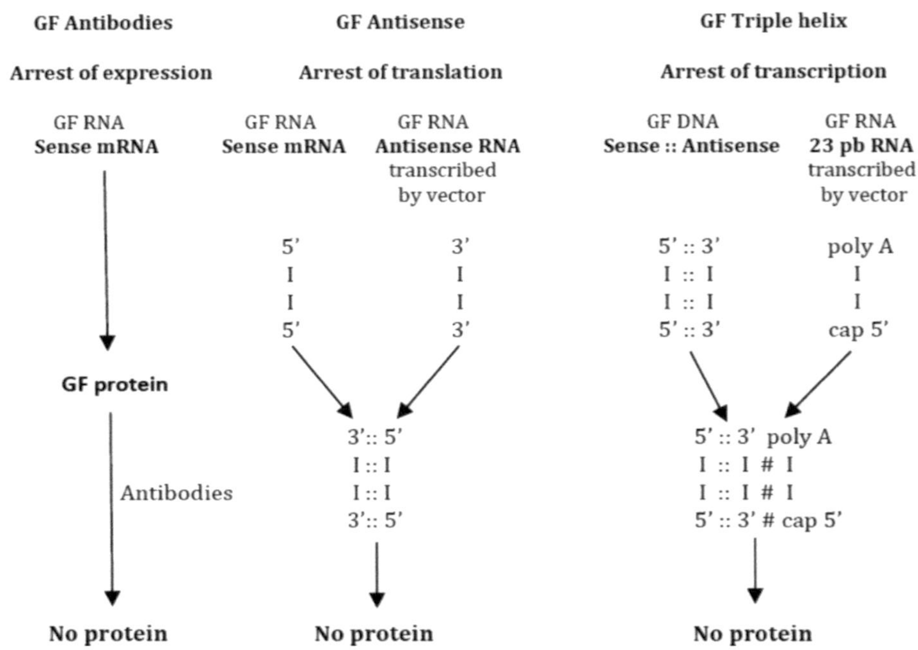

Figure 1.
Schema of technologies suppressing the expression of oncoproteins, including growth factors, GF: antibodies, antisense and triple helix. In antibodies technology, the GF expression is directly blocked by its ligand—antibody. In antisense technology, the end result is the inhibition of GF mRNA (sense RNA) activity by binding to the antisense RNA. In triple helix technology, the oligopurine third strand (23 bp) forms RNA-DNA triple helix with GF gene.

3.2 Antisense and triple helix experimental studies

In our experimental studies, we have shown that in IGF-I "antisense" and "triple helix" transfected CNS-1 rat glioma cells, PCC-4 mouse embryonal carcinoma cells, and in primary human glioma cells, changes in immunogenic properties and apoptosis occur. The induction of IGF-I triple helix forming structure, similarly to IGF-I antisense approach, was followed by enhanced expression of MHC-I and B-7 [5, 18, 90–95] and loss of *in vivo* tumorigenicity. An extensive lymphocytic CD8 positive infiltration 4–5 days after injection of AS transfected glioma, teratocarcinoma and hepatoma cells into the respective animal bearing tumors was demonstrated [11, 27, 96]. These properties were used for selection of human glioma cells that were used in IGF-I antisense/triple helix immunogene therapy [90] (**Figure 2**).

In this context, antigenic peptides presented by class I MHC molecules were necessary but, in general, not sufficient to stimulate T cell response. In the absence of B-7 molecule, MHC-peptide complexes could selectively inactivate T-cells [97]. (Although "triple helix" cells as compared to "antisense" cells show slightly higher expression of MHC-I and B7 there are no qualitative immunogenic and apoptotic differences between IGF-I "antisense" and "triple helix" approaches).

The absence of IGF-I synthesis in AS and TH transfected cells, could lead to a higher level of IGF-I receptor and hence to greater tyrosine kinase content [98]. There is a relation between the signal transduction pathway of tyrosine kinase and induction of B-7 molecules: enhancement in B-7 co-stimulation through a cAMP mechanism linked to tyrosine kinase of the CD 28 receptor has been previously reported [99]. Similar signaling through the tyrosine kinase activity of the IGF-I receptor shows that: tyrosine kinase activates IRS-1 (Insulin receptor substrate-1),

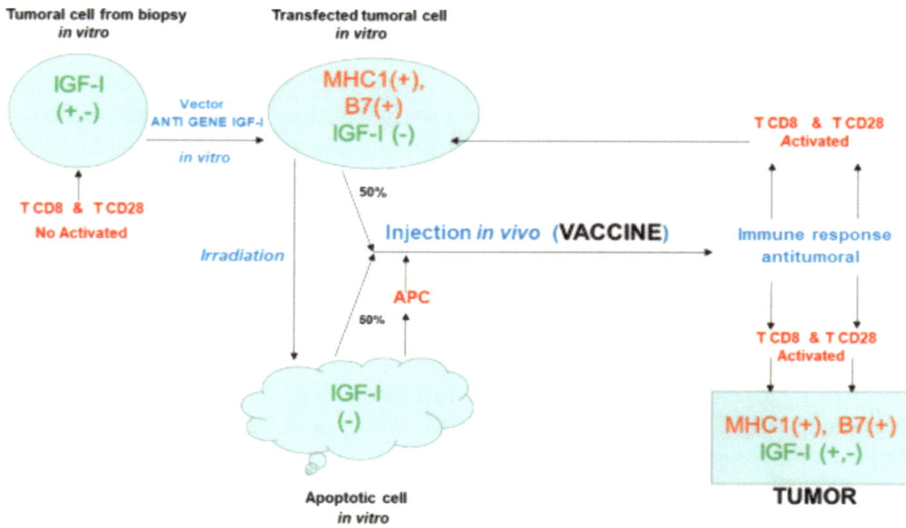

Figure 2.
Schema of cancer immunogene therapy. The cells isolated from tumor biopsy are growing in tissue culture. The established cell line is transfected by vector of anti-gene type (antisense and triple helix IGF-I). The transfected cells, and originated apoptotic cells, are injected in proportion 50–50 ("vaccine") in the cancer patients. The presence of MHC-I and B7 molecules present in transfected tumor cells induce an immune response mediated by T lymphocytes. Moreover, APC cells also participate as shown in the immunogene mechanism. The activated T lymphocytes destroy as well the vaccine (transfected tumor cells) as a tumor.

and then IRS-1 activates PI3K (phosphatidylinositol 3 kinase) [100, 101]. This mechanism could be considered in the cytokine induced B7–1 expression demonstrated in fetal human microglia in culture [102].

In the AS and TH transfected cells, IGF-I-R activated by its ligand plays a very protective role in programmed cell death, and that this protection is even more striking *in vivo* than *in vitro* [103]. Apoptosis could play a specific role in our strategies; the phenotypic modifications due to apoptosis may explain the recognition of the transfected cells by the immune system like tumor-specific immunity mediated by CD8+ T [11, 98]. Apoptotic cells, in the context of MHC-I are recognized by dendritic cells activating lymphocytes T-CD8 [104, 105]. B-7 molecules can be included in this mechanism, because both MHC-I and B-7 molecules are necessary for T cell activation [16, 27, 36, 91, 106–108].

While working on mouse hepatoma cells transfected by the IGF-I triple helix approach, we have observed a decrease of cytokines such as Il-10, which is a strong immunosuppressor [109], and TNF-alpha, which can act as a factor stimulating tumor growth [110, 111]. Moreover, we have found increased levels of TAP 1 and 2 in these cells. The relationship between the immune process, related to the MHC-I or HLA system [112, 113], and the apoptotic process is under study.

3.3 Anti-gene clinical therapy

In the clinical trial using anti-gene IGF-I therapy after subcutaneous vaccination, the subject developed peri-tumor necrosis; the tissue section bordering the necrotic tumor tissue showed infiltration of lymphocytes consisting of both CD4 and CD8 T cells [114]. Other results concerning peripheral blood lymphocytes (PBL) of glioblastoma patients treated by IGF-I triple helix immuno-gene therapy show eminent changes in CD8 T cells, especially after second injection. There was also an increase in the percentage of CD8 with characteristics switching from CD8+

CD11b+ to CD8+ CD11b− phenotype, an alteration that may reflect the enhanced activation of T cytotoxic cells in blood. Additionally, as far as prognosis of glioblastoma patients is concerned, the patients have survived between 18 and 24 months after the first diagnosis. Generally, patients with diagnosed glioblastoma multiforme, undergoing surgeries and radiotherapy, survive up to 14 months [22, 113].

Our phase I human cancer clinical trial based on the anti-gene, antisense approach, is in progress in the U.S.A, Thailand, Poland and China [107, 114, 115] and is in parallel with previously established approaches of glioblastoma treatment established by either Culver [116] or by Baserga [65]. Following the same approach, different antisense strategies to treat glioma tumors have been recently investigated [26, 31, 117, 118], especially in relation to glycogen metabolism [119] in glioma cells. (Malignant astrocytes present a high level of glycogen [55]). The therapy of gliomas using strategies of growth factors inhibition is in permanent progress. The inhibition of the IGF-I receptor using AS technology, and its signaling pathway has opened a door for experimental and clinical research in various tumors [9, 14, 15, 42, 62, 120, 121].

4. Discussion

The use of anti-gene therapy was also effective in another AS approach, targeted toward the molecule, TGF-beta [79]. TGF-beta2 plays a role in tumor progression by regulating key mechanisms including proliferation, metastasis, and angiogenesis. The approach of AS TGF-beta using an AS oligodeoxynucleotide—compound AP 12009, has given satisfactory results [122–124]. AP-12009 treatment was well tolerated and tumor response has been observed [123]. Two patients experienced long-lasting complete tumor remission [124]. In another clinical AS TGF-beta study, a phase I clinical trial in grade IV astrocytoma (GBM) was performed using autologous tumor cells modified by a AS TGF-beta2 vector [79]. There were indications of humoral and cellular immunity induced by the vaccine [57, 79].

As far as AS TGF-beta therapy of GBM is concerned, the treatment of patients with recurrent or refractory malignant (high-grade) glioma, WHO grade III or IV has been shown to produce results, similar to results obtained with anti IGF-I treatment. The role of peripheral blood mononuclear cells in the immune antitumor response, and prolonged survival in both anti TGF beta and anti IGF-I approaches was comparatively examined. In the case of TGF-beta, it is also important to mention, that although the first successful clinical results were published in 2006–2008, the solid experimental data, using AS technology were obtained in 1994/95 [79], which means, that long periods of research on the mechanism of AS TGF-beta and AS IGF I are required before achieving significant clinical results, confirming the usefulness of gene therapy in cancer treatment [90, 122, 123, 125–130].

In AS IGF-I or AS TGF-beta approaches, immune antitumor response, mediated by TCD8 and APC cells, was signaled as a principal mechanism of AS technology inhibiting growth factors and their signaling pathway [12, 79]. These cells being involved in HS (heat shock) protein mechanism, the inhibition of HS was introduced in clinical trials as a new direction for cancer therapy [131].

More recent clinical successful strategies of gliomas treatment, generally as a combination therapy using different types of inhibitors (i.e., imatinib, gefitinib) including antibodies (i.e., avastin) targeting growth factors and their receptors [132–136], are now focusing on anti-gene strategy, especially on antisense or triple helix technologies used alone or combined also with pharmacological treatment. As far as antisense and triple helix strategies are compared, the triple helix blockade of growth factor has given better results *in vitro* and *in vivo*. But combining both strategies, the final result is most effective—stopping the expression of the oncoproteins on translation (AS) and transcription (TH) levels, respectively.

5. Conclusion

Among the new strategies in the efforts to successfully treat GBM, the use of AS approach targeting IGF-I, TGF-beta or VEGF, their receptors and their downstream transduction signaling elements [9, 137], appears to offer a promising solution. The final result of the signal transduction pathway element inhibition is an immune response mediated *in vivo* by lymphocytes T CD8 and APC cells. Using cancer immunogene therapy of anti-gene anti IGF-I approach, the median survival of treated glioblastoma patients has reached 22–24 months. But the near future in treating this group of disorders belongs to a combination of treatment: classical surgery, radiotherapy with immunotherapy, pharmacologic therapy, growth factor inhibitors, and the use of the antisense/triple helix gene blockade approach targeting signal transduction pathway elements of cancer processes [16, 22, 23, 36, 66, 90, 125, 138–147].

Conflict of interest

No conflict of interest.

Author details

Jerzy Trojan[1,2,3,4*]

1 Laboratories Legrand, Bogota, Colombia

2 ICGT–International Cancer Gene Therapy, Bogota, Colombia

3 ICGT–International Cancer Gene Therapy, Paris, France

4 INSERM, Paris, France

*Address all correspondence to: genetherapy@hotmail.fr

IntechOpen

© 2019 The Author(s). Licensee IntechOpen. This chapter is distributed under the terms of the Creative Commons Attribution License (http://creativecommons.org/licenses/by/3.0), which permits unrestricted use, distribution, and reproduction in any medium, provided the original work is properly cited.

References

[1] Abelev GJ. Alpha-fetoprotein in ontogenesis and its association with malignant tumors. Advances in Cancer Research. 1971;**14**:295-299

[2] Trojan J, Uriel J, Deugnier MA, Gaillard J. Immunocytochemical quantitative study of alphafetoprotein in normal and neoplastic neural development. Developmental Neuroscience. 1984;**6**:251-259

[3] Hajeri-Germond M, Naval J, Trojan J, et al. The uptake of alphafetoprotein by C-1300 mouse neuroblastoma cells. British Journal of Cancer. 1985;**51**:791-797

[4] Trojan J, Naval X, Johnson T, et al. Expression of serum albumin and of alphafetoprotein in murine normal and neoplastic primitive embryonic structures of teratocarcinoma. Molecular Reproduction and Development. 1995;**42**(4):369-378

[5] Harding BN, Golden JA. Developmental Neuropathology. Basel, Switzerland: International Society of Neuropathology; 2004

[6] Calaminus G, Bamberg M, Harms D, et al. AFP/β-HCG secreting CNS germ cell tumors: Long-term outcome with respect to initial symptoms and primary tumor resection. Results of the Cooperative Trial MAKEI 89. Neuropediatrics. 2005;**36**(2):71-77

[7] Kim A, Ji L, Balmaceda C, et al. The prognostic value of tumor markers in newly diagnosed patients with primary central nervous system germ cell tumors. Pediatric Blood & Cancer. 2008;**51**(6):768-773

[8] Kawaguchi T, Kumabe T, Kanamori M, et al. Logarithmic decrease of serum alpha-fetoprotein or human chorionic gonadotropin in response to chemotherapy can distinguish a subgroup with better prognosis among highly malignant intracranial non-germinomatous germ cell tumors. Journal of Neurooncology. 2011;**104**(3):779-787

[9] Trojan J, Cloix J-F, Ardourel M, et al. IGF-I biology and targeting in malignant glioma. Neuroscience. 2007;**145**(3):795-811

[10] Kiess W, Lee L, Graham DE, et al. Rat C6 glial cells synthesize insulin-like growth factor I (IGF-I) and express IGF-I re-ceptors and IGF-II/mannose 6-phosphate re-ceptors. Endocrinology. 1989;**124**:1727-1736

[11] Trojan J, Johnson T, Rudin S, et al. Treatment and prevention of rat glioblastoma by immugenic C6 cells expressing antisense insulin-like growth factor I RNA. Science. 1993;**259**:94-97

[12] Ly A, Duc HT, Kalamarides M, et al. Human glioma cells transformed by IGF-I tri-ple-helix technology show immune and apoptotic characteristics determining cell selection for gene therapy of glioblastoma. Journal of Clinical Pathology (Molecular Pathology). 2001;**54**:230-239

[13] Zumkeller W. IGFs and IGF-binding proteins as diagnostic markers and biological modulators in brain tumors. Expert Review of Molecular Diagnostics. 2002;**2**:473-477

[14] Pollak MN, Schernhammer ES, Hankinson SE. Insulin-like growth factors and neoplasia. Nature Reviews. Cancer. 2004;**4**:505-518. DOI: 10.1038/nrc1387

[15] Baserga R. The insulin-like growth factor-I receptor as a target for cancer therapy. Expert Opinion on Therapeutic Targets. 2005;**9**:753-768

[16] Pan Y, Trojan J, Guo Y, et al. Rescue of MHC-1 antigen processing machinery by down-regulation in expression of IGF-I in human glioblastoma cells. PLoS One. 2013;**8**(3):e58428. DOI: 10.1371/0058428

[17] Trojan A, Jay LM, Briceño I, et al. IGF-I, IGF-I gene and diagnostic. In: Trojan J, editor. Cancer Immunogene Therapy. Anti-Gene Anti IGF-I Approach. Case of Glioblastoma. Saarbrucken, Germany: Lambert Academic Publishers; 2017. pp. 7-28. ISBN-13: 978-3-330-06345-7; ISBN-10: 3330063459

[18] Trojan J, Blossey BK, Johnson T, et al. Loss of tumorogenicity of rat glioblastoma directed by episome-based antisense cDNA transcription of insulin-like growth factor I. Proceedings of the National Academy of Sciences of the United States of America. 1992;**89**(11):4874-4878

[19] Le Roith D, Bondy C, Yakar S, Liu JL, Butler A. The somatomedin hypothesis. Endocrine Reviews. 2011;**22**(1):53-74. DOI: 10.1210/edrv.22.1.0419

[20] Froesch CS, Schwander J, Zapf J. Actions of insulin-like growth factors. Annual Review of Physiology. 1985;**47**:443-467

[21] Johnson TR, Trojan J, Rudin SD, et al. Effects on actinomycin D and cycloheximide on transcript levels of IGF- I, actin and albumin in hepatocyte primary cultures treated with growth hormone and insulin. Molecular Reproduction and Development. 1991;**30**:95-99

[22] Trojan A, Jay LM, Kasprzak H, et al. Immunotherapy of malignant tumors using antisense anti-IGF-I approach: Case of glioblastoma. Journal of Cancer Therapy. 2014;**5**:685-705

[23] Trojan J. Anti – Gene anti IGF-I technology applied for cancer immunotherapy. World Journal of Research Review. 2016;**1**(3):67-75

[24] Trojan J, Uriel J. Immunocytochemical signaling of alpha fetoprotein (AFP) and serum-albumin (Alb) in ecto-, mesa- and endodermal tissue derivatives of the developing rat. Oncodevelopmental Biology and Medicine. 1982;**3**:12-22

[25] Benno RH, Williams TH. Evidence for intracellular localization of AFP in the developing rat brain. Brain Research. 1978;**142**:182-186

[26] Trojan J, Uriel J. Localisation intracellulaire of l'AFP et de la serum albumine dans le fœtal nerveux central du rat au cours du developpement fœtal et postnatal. Comptes Rendus de l'Académie des Sciences Paris. 1979;**289**:1157-1160

[27] Trojan J, Johnson TR, Rudin SD, et al. Gene therapy of murine teratocarcinoma: Separate functions for insulin-like growth factors I and II in immunogenicity and differentiation. Proceedings of the National Academy of Sciences of the United States of America. 1994;**91**:6088-6092

[28] Schubert D, Humphreys S, Baroni C, Cohn M. In vitro differentiation of a mouse neuroblastoma. Biochemistry. 1969;**64**:316-323

[29] Bernal S, Thompson RA, Gilbert F, Baylin S. In vitro and in vivo growth characteristics of two different cell populations in an established line of human neuroblastoma. Cancer Research. 1983;**43**:125-164

[30] Uriel J, Faivre-Baumann A, Trojan J, et al. Immunocytochemical demonstration of alphafoetoprotein uptake by primary cultures of foetal

hemisphere cells from mouse brain. Neuroscience Letters. 1981;**27**:171-175

[31] Uriel J, Poupon MF, Geuskens M. Alphaignaling uptake by cloned cell lines derived from a nickel-induced rat rhabdomyosarcoma. British Journal of Cancer. 1983;**48**:261-269

[32] Uriel J, Villacampa MJ, Moro R, et al. Uptake of radiolabeled alphafetoprotein by mouse mammary carcinomas and usefulness in tumor scientigraphy. Cancer Research. 1984;**44**:5314-5319

[33] Gaillard J, Caillaud JM, Maunoury R, et al. Expression du neuroectoblaste dans le teratocarcinome et le teratome de la souris. Bulletin de l'Institut Pasteur. 1984;**82**:335-385

[34] Trojan J, Uriel J, Gaillard JA. Localisation de alphafoetoproteine dans les derives neuroepitheliaux des teratocarcinomes de la souris. Annales de Pathologie. 1983;**3**:137-145

[35] Hajeri-Germond M, Trojan J, Uriel J, et al. In vitro uptake of exogenous alphafetoprotein by chicken dorsal root ganglia. Developmental Neuroscience. 1984;**6**:111-117

[36] Castillo T, Trojan A, Noguera MC, et al. Epistemiologic experience in elaboration of molecular biology technology for immunogene therapy (in Spanish). Revista Cientifica. 2016;**2**:25. DOI: 10.14483/udistrital.jour.RC.2016.25.a6

[37] Benedetti E, Galzio R, D'Angelo B, et al. PPARs in human neuroepithelial tumors: PPAR ligands as anticancer therapies for the most common human neuroepithelial tumors. PPAR Research. 2010:401-427. DOI: 10.1155/2010/427401

[38] Lichtor T. Evolution of the Molecular Biology of Brain Tumors and the Therapeutic Implications. Vienna/Rijeka: InTech; 2013

[39] Love S, Arie Perry A, Ironside J, Budka H. Greenfield's Neuropathology. 9th ed. New York: CRC Press; 2015

[40] Daughaday WH, Hall K, Raben MS, et al. Somatomedin: Proposed designation for sulphation factor. Nature. 1972;**235**:107

[41] Han VKM, Hill DJ. In: Shofield PN, editor. The Insulin-Like Growth Factors: Structure and Biological Functions. Oxford, England: Oxford University Press; 1992. pp. 178-219

[42] Baserga R, Sell C, Porcu P, Rubini M. The role of the IGF-I receptor in the growth and transformation of mammalian cells. Cell Proliferation. 1994;**27**:63-71

[43] Baserga R. Oncogenes and the strategy of growth factors. Cell. 1994;**79**:927-930

[44] Sturm MA, Conover CA, Pham H, et al. Insulin like growth factor receptors and binding proteins in rat neuroblastoma. Endocrinology. 1989;**124**:388-396

[45] Werther GA, Abate M, Hogg A, et al. Localisation of Insulin like growth factor mRNA in rat brain by in situ hybridization-relation to IGF-I rceceptor. Molecular Endocrinology. 1990;**4**:773-778

[46] Antoniades HN, Galanopoulis T, Nevile-Golden J, et al. Expression of insulin like growth factor I and II and their receptor mRNAs in primary human astrocytomas and meningiomas: In vivo studies using in situ hybridization and immunocytochemistry. International Journal of Cancer. 1992;**50**:215-222

[47] Trojan J, Uriel J, Deugnier MA, et al. Immunocytochemical quantitative study of alpha-fetoprotein in normal and neoplastic neural development. Developmental Neuroscience.

1984;**6**(4-5):251-259. DOI: 10.1159/000112352

[48] Ostos H, Astaiza G, Garcia F, et al. Decreased incidence of defects of neural tube closure at the University Hospital of Neiva: Possible effect promotion of folic acid (in Spanish). Biomédica. 2000;**20**(1):18-24. DOI: 10.7705/ignaling.v20i1.1043

[49] Le Roith D. The insulin-like growth factor system. Experimental Diabesity Research. 2003;**4**(4):205-212. DOI: 10.1155/EDR.2003.205

[50] Adhami VM, Afaq F, Mukhtar H. Insulin-like growth factor-I axis as a pathway for cancer chemoprevention. Clinical Cancer Research. 2006;**12**(19):5611-5614. DOI: 10.1158/1078-0432.CCR-06-1564

[51] Chen H, Mester T, Raychaudhuri N, et al. Teprotumumab, an IGF-1R blocking monoclonal antibody inhibits TSH and IGF-1 action in fibrocytes. Journal of Clinical Endocrinology and Metabolism. 2014;**99**(9):E1635-E1640. DOI: 10.1210/jc.2014-1580

[52] Kooijman R. Regulation of apoptosis by insulin-like growth factor (IGF)-I. Cytokine & Growth Factor Reviews. 2006;**17**(4):305-323. DOI: 10.1016/j.cytogfr.2006.02.002

[53] Bueno S, Santandr R, Alvarez A, et al. Brain stem cells and IGF-I: Implications in development, regeneration and cancer therapeutics. Integrative Molecular Medicine. 2018;**5**(1). DOI: 10.15761/IMM.1000319

[54] Kurmasheva RT, Houghton PJ. IGF-I mediated survival pathways in normal and malignant cells. Biochimica et Biophysica Acta. 2006;**1766**(1):1-22. DOI: 10.1016/j.bbcan.2006.05.003

[55] Beckner ME, Gobbel GT, Abounader R, et al. Glycolytic glioma cells with active glycogen synthase are sensitive to PTEN and inhibitors of PI3K and gluconeogenesis. Laboratory Investigation. 2005;**85**(12):1457-1470. DOI: 10.1038/labinvest.3700355

[56] Vignot S, Faivre S, Aguirre D, et al. mTOR-targeted therapy of cancer with rapamycin derivatives. Annals of Oncology. 2005;**16**(4):525-537

[57] Schlingensiepen KH, Jaschinski F, Lang SA, et al. Transforming growth factor-beta 2 gene silencing with trabedersen (AP 12009) in pancreatic cancer. Cancer Science. 2011;**102**(6):1193-1200. DOI: 10.1111/j.1349-7006.2011.01917.x

[58] Trojan J, Anthony DD. Antisense strategies in therapy of gliomas. Current Signal Transduction Therapy. 2011;**6**(3):411-423. DOI: 10.2174/157436211797483895

[59] Patel S, Doble B, Woodgett JR. Glycogen synthase kinase-3 in insulin and Wnt signaling: A double-edged sword? Biochemical Society - Translation UK. 2004;**32**(5):803-808. DOI: 10.1042/BST0320803

[60] Jiang R, Mircean C, Shmulevich I, et al. Pathway alterations during glioma progression revealed by reverse phase protein lysate arrays. Proteomics. 2006;**6**(10):2964-2971. DOI: 10.1002/pmic.200500555

[61] Hutterer M, Gunsilius E, Stockhammer G. Molecular therapies for malignant glioma. Wien Medicinal Wochenschreibung. 2006;**156**(11):351-363. DOI: 10.1007/s10354-006-0308-3

[62] Sachdev D, Yee D. Disrupting insulin-like growth factor signaling as a potential cancer therapy. Molecular Cancer Therapy. 2007;**6**(1):1-12. DOI: 10.1158/1535-7163.MCT-06-0080

[63] Ardourel M, Blin M, Moret JL, et al. A new putative target for antisense gene therapy of glioma: Glycogen synthetase.

Cancer Biology and Therapy. 2007;**6**(5):719-723. DOI: 10.4161/cbt.6.5.4232

[64] Zhou X, Ren Y, Moore L, et al. Downregulation of miR-21 inhibits EGFR pathway and suppresses the growth of human glioblastoma cells independent of PTEN status. Laboratory Investigation. 2010;**90**:144-155. DOI: 10.1038/labinvest.2009.126

[65] Premkumar DR, Arnold B, Jane EP, et al. Synergistic interaction between 17-AAG and phosphatidylinositol 3-kinase inhibition in human malignant glioma cells. Molecular Carcinogenesis. 2006;**45**(1):47-59. DOI: 10.1002/mc.20152

[66] Sanson M, Laigle-Donadey F, Benouaich-Amiel A. Molecular changes in brain tumours: Prognostic and therapeutic impact. Current Opinion in Oncology. 2006;**18**(6):623-630. DOI: 10.1097/01.cco.0000245322.11787.72

[67] Trojan J, Briceno I. IGF-I antisense and triple-helix gene therapy of glioblastoma. In: Pantar A, editor. Evolution of the Molecular Biology of Brain Tumors and the Therapeutic Implications. Vienna/Rijeka: InTech; 2013. pp. 149-166

[68] Esiri M, Perl D. Oppenheimer's Diagnostic Neuropathology. 3rd ed. FL: CRC Press; 2006

[69] Glick RP, Lichtor T, Unterman TG. Insulin-like growth factors in central nervous system tumors. Journal of Neuro-Oncology. 1997;**35**(3):315-325

[70] Obrepalska-Steplowska A, Kedzia A, Trojan J, et al. Analysis of coding and promoter sequences of the IGF-I gene in children with growth disorders presenting with normal level of growth hormone. Journal of Pediatric Endocrinology and Metabolism. 2003;**16**(9):1267-1275

[71] Hu B, Niu X, Cheng L, et al. Discovering cancer biomarkers from clinical samples by protein microarrays. Proteomics: Clinical Applications. 2015;**9**(1-2):98-110. DOI: 10.1002/prca.201400094

[72] Ertl DA, Gleiss A, Sagmeister S, et al. Determining the normal range for IGF-I, IGFBP-3, and ALS: New reference data based on current internal standards. Wiener Medizinische Wochenschrift. 2014;**164**(17-18):343-352. DOI: 10.1007/sl 0354-014-0299-4

[73] Gu F, Schumacher FR, Canzian F, et al. Eighteen insulin-like growth factor pathway genes, circulating levels of IGF-I and its binding protein, and risk of prostate and breast cancer. Cancer Epidemiology, Biomarkers & Prevention. 2010;**19**(11):2877-2887. DOI: 10.1158/1055-9965.EPI-10-0507

[74] Mosquera CJ, Castelblanco OL. Didactic questions and epistemiology (in Spanish). Revista Gondola. 2015;**10**(1). DOI: 10.14483/udistrital.jour.GDLA.2015.1.a00

[75] Stupp R, Hegi ME, van den Bent MJ, et al. Changing paradigms—An update on the multidisciplinary management of malignant glioma. The Oncologist. 2006;**11**:165-180

[76] Kjaergaard J, Wang L, Kuriyama H, Shu S, Plautz GE. Active immunotherapy for advanced intracranial murine tumors by using dendritic cell-tumor cell fusion vaccines. Journal of Neurosurgery. 2005;**103**:156-164

[77] Rubenstein JL, Nicolas JF, Jacob F. Nonsense RNA: A tool for specifically inhibiting the expression of a gene in vivo. Comptes Rendus de l'Académie des Sciences, Paris III. 1984;**299**:271-274

[78] Weintraub H, Izant J, Harland R. Antisense RNA as a molecular tool

for genetic analysis. Trends in Genetics. 1985;**1**(1):23-25

[79] Fakhrai H, Dorigo O, Shawler DL, et al. Eradication of established intracranial rat gliomas by transforming growth factor beta antisense gene therapy. Proceedings of the National Academy of Sciences of the United States of America. 1996;**93**(7):2909-2914

[80] Dervan P. Reagents for the sitespecific cleavage of megabase DNA. Nature. 1992;**359**:87-88

[81] Hélène C. Control of oncogene expression by antisense nucleic acid. European Journal of Cancer. 1994;**30A**:1721-1726

[82] Berezikov E, Thuemmler F, van Laake LW, et al. Diversity of microRNAs in human and chimpanzee brain. Nature Genetics. 2006;**38**(12):1375-1377

[83] Corsten MF, Miranda R, Kasmieh R, et al. MicroRNA-21 knockdown disrupts glioma growth in vivo and displays synergistic cytotoxicity with neural precursor cell delivered S-TRAIL in human gliomas. Cancer Research. 2007;**67**(19):8994-9000

[84] Boado RJ. RNA interference and nonviral targeted gene therapy of experimental brain cancer. NeuroRx. 2005;**2**(1):139-150

[85] Paï SI, Lin YY, Macaes B, et al. Prospects of RNA interference therapy for cancer. Gene Therapy. 2006;**13**(6):464-477

[86] Shevelev A, Burfeind P, Schulze E, et al. Potential triple helix mediated inhibition of IGF-I gene expression significantly reduces tumorigenicity of glioblastoma in an animal model. Cancer Gene Therapy. 1997;**4**:105-112

[87] Rininsland F, Johnson T, Chernicky C, et al. Suppression of insulin-like growth factor type-I receptor by a triple-helix strategy inhibits IGF-I transcription and tumorigenic potential of rat C6 glioblastoma cells. Proceedings of the National Academy of Sciences of the United States of America. 1997;**94**:5854-5859

[88] Dias N, Stein CA. Basic concepts and antisense oligonucleotides mechanisms. Molecular Cancer Therapeutics. 2002;**1**:347-355

[89] Wells DJ. Therapeutic restoration of dystrophin expression in Duchenne muscular dystrophy. Journal of Muscle Research and Cell Motility. 2006;**27**(5-7):387-398

[90] Trojan J, Pan YX, Wei MX, et al. Methodology for anti-gene anti-IGF-I therapy of malignant tumours. Chemotherapy Research and Practice. 2011/2012. DOI: 10.1155/2012/721873

[91] Townsend SE, Allison JA. Tumor rejection after direct costi-mulation of CD8+ T cell transfected melanoma cells. Science 1993;259: 368-370

[92] Guo Y, Wu M, Chen H, et al. Effective tumor vaccine generated by fusion of hepatoma cells with lymphocytes B cells. Science. 1994;**263**:518-520

[93] Trojan J. Cancer Immunogene Therapy. Anti-Gene Anti IGF-I Approach. Case of Glioblastoma. Germany: Lambert Academic Publishers; 2017. 140p. ISBN-13: 978-3-330-06345-7; ISBN-10: 3330063459

[94] Linsley PS, Clark EA, Ledbetter JA. T-cell antigen CD28 mediates adhesion with B cells by interacting with ativation antigen B7/13. Proceedings of the National Academy of Sciences of the United States of America. 1990;**87**:5031-5035

[95] Freeman GB, Gray GS, Gimmi CD, et al. Structure

[96] Upegui-Gonzalez LC, Ly A, Sierzega M, et al. IGF-I triple helix strategy in hepatoma treatment. Hepato-Gastroenterology. 2001;**48**:660-666

[97] Steiman RM, Turkey S, Mellman I, Inaba K. The induction of tolerance by dendritic cells that have captured apoptotic cells. Journal of Experimental Medicine. 2000;**191**:411-416

[98] Lafarge-Frayssinet C, Sarasin A, Duc HT, et al. Gene therapy for hepatocarcinoma: Antisense IGF-I transfer into a rat hepatoma cell line inhibits tumorigenesis into syngeneic animal. Cancer Gene Therapy. 1997;**4**:276-285

[99] Schwartz RH. Costimulation of T lymphocytes: The role of CD28, CTLA-4 and B7/BBI in interleukin-2 production and immunotherapy. Cell. 1992;**71**:1065-1068

[100] D'Ambrosio C, Ferber A, Resnicoff M, et al. A soluble insulin-like growth factor receptor that induces apoptosis of tumor cells in vivo and inhibits tumorigenesis. Cancer Research. 1996;**56**:4013-4020

[101] Dudek H, Datta SR, Franke TS, et al. Regulation of neuronal servival by the serine-threonine protein kinase. Akta Science. 1997;**275**:661-665

[102] Satoh J, Lee YB, Kim SU. T-cell costimulatory molecules B7-1 (CD80) and B7-2 (CD86) are expressed in human microglia but not in astrocytes in culture. Brain Research. 1995;**704**:95-96

[103] Resnicoff M, Abraham D, Yutanawiboonchai W, et al. The insulin-like growth factor I receptor protects tumor cells from apoptosis in vitro. Cancer Research. 1995;**55**:2463-2469

[104] Sotomayor E, Fu Y, Lopez-Cepero M, et al. Role of tumor derived cytokines on the immune system of mice bearing a mammary adenocarcinoma. Journal of Immunology. 1991;**147**:2816-2823

[105] Matthew L, Saiter B, Bhardwag N. Dendritic cells acquire antigen from apoptotic cells and induce class I restricted CTL. Nature. 1998;**392**:86-89

[106] Chen L, Ashe S, Brady WA, et al. Costimulation of anti-tumor immunity by the B7 counter receptor for the T lymphocyte molecules CD28 and CTLA-4. Cell. 1992;**71**:1093-1102

[107] Anthony D, Pan Y, Wu S, et al. Ex vivo and in vivo IGF-I antisense RNA strategies for treatment of cancer in humans. Advances in Experimental Medicine and Biology. 1998;**451**:27-34

[108] Zhu C, Trabado S, Fan Y, et al. Characterization of effector components from the humoral and cellular immune response stimulated by melanoma cells exhibiting modified IGF-1 expression. Biomedicine & Pharmacotherapy. 2015;**70**:53-57. DOI: 10.1016/j.biopha.2015.01.002

[109] Gerard CM, Bruyns C, Delvaux A, et al. Loss of tumorigenicity and increased immunogenicity induced by interleukin-10 gene transfer in B16 melanoma cells. Human Gene Therapy. 1996;**7**(1):23-31

[110] Buck C, Digel W, Schoniger W, et al. Tumor nercrosis factor alpha but not lymphotoxin, stimulates growth of tumor cells in hairy cell leukemia. Leukemia. 1990;**4**:431-439

[111] Aggarwal B, Schwarz L, Hogan M, et al. Triple helixforming oligodeoxiribonucleotides targeted to the human tumor necrosis factor (TNF) gene inhibit TNF production and block the TNF dependent growth of human glioblastoma tumor cells. Cancer Research. 1996;**56**:5156-5164

[112] Blanchet O, Bourge JF, Zinszner H, et al. Altered binding of regulatory factors to HLA class I enhancer sequence in human tumor cell lines lacking class I antigen expression. Proceedings of the National Academy of Sciences of the United States of America. 1992;**89**(8):3488-3492

[113] Trojan LA, Ly A, Kopinski P, et al. Antisense and triple helix anti IGF-I tumour vaccines: Gene therapy of gliomas. International Journal of Cancer Prevention. 2007;**2**(4):227-243

[114] Wongkajornslip A, Ouyprasertkul M, Sangruchi T, et al. The analysis of peri-tumor necrosis following the subcutaneous implantation of autologous tumor cells transfected with an episome transcribing an antisense insulin-like growth factor I RNA in a glioblastoma multiforme subject. Journal of the Medical Association of Thailand. 2001;**m4**(3):740-747

[115] Trojan LA, Kopinski P, Mazurek A, et al. IGF I triple helix gene therapy of rat and human gliomas. Annales Academiae Medicae Bialostocensis. 2003;**48**:18-27

[116] Culver KW, Rarn Z, Wallbridge S. In vivo gene transfer with retroviral vector-producer cells for treatment of experimental brain tumors. Science. 1992;**256**:1550-1552

[117] Kopinski P, Ly A, Trojan J. Chapter 44: Antisense in oncology. In: Khayat D, Ly A, editors. About Cancer in Africa. Paris, France: Springer; 2005/2006

[118] Grossman SA, Alavi JB, Supko JG, et al. Efficacy and toxicity of the antisense oligonucleotide aprinocarsen directed against protein kinase C-alpha delivered as a 21-day continuous intravenous infusion in patients with recurrent high-grade astrocytomas. Neuro-Oncology. 2005;**7**(1):32-40

[119] Bernard-Helary K, Ardourel M, Magistrett P, et al. Stable transfection of cDNAs targeting specific steps of glycogen metabolism supports the existence of active gluconeogenesis in mouse cultured astrocytes. Glia. 2002;**37**(4):379-382

[120] Andrews DW, Resnicoff M, Flanders A, et al. Results of a pilot study involving the use of an antisense oligodeoxynucleotide directed against the insulin-like growth factor type I receptor in malignant astrocytomas. Journal of Clinical Oncology. 2001;**19**:2189-2200

[121] Samani AA, Fallavollita L, Jaalouk DE, et al. Inhibition of carcinoma cell growth and metastasis by a vesicular stomatitis virus G-pseudotyped retrovector expressing type 1 insulin-like growth factor receptor antisense. Human Gene Therapy. 2001;**12**:1969-1977

[122] Schlingensiepen R, Goldbrunner M, Szyrach MNI, et al. Intracerebral and intrathecal infusion of the TGF-beta2-specific antisense phosphorothioate oligonucleotide AP 12009 in rabbits and primates: Toxicology and safety. Oligonucleotides. 2005;**15**(2):94-104

[123] Schlingensiepen KH, Schlingensiepen R, Steinbrecher A, et al. Targeted tumor therapy with the TGF-beta2 antisense compound AP 12009. Cytokine & Growth Factor Reviews. 2006;**17**:129-139

[124] Hau P, Jachimczak P, Schlingensiepen R, et al. Inhibition of TGF-beta2 with AP 12009 in recurrent malignant gliomas: From preclinical to phase I/II studies. Oligonucleotides. 2007;**17**(2):201-212

[125] Schlingensiepen KH, Fischer-Blass B, Schmaus S, et al. Antisense therapeutics for tumor treatment: the TGF-beta2 inhibitor AP 12009 in

clinical development against malignant tumors. Recent Results in Cancer Research. 2008;**177**:137-150

[126] Anthony DD. Ex vivo and in vivo IGF-1 antisense RNA strategies for treatment of cancers in humans [Abstract]. Cancer Gene Therapy. 1997;**2**(6):S322

[127] Popiela T, Sierzega M, Gach T, et al. Phase I trial of colorectal cancer immunotherapy using autologous cancer cells transfected with an IGF-I antisense plasmid [abstract]. Acta Chirurgica Belgica. 2003;**5**(103):S2-S3

[128] Schlingensiepen R, Goldbrunner M, Bischof A, et al. Antisense-TGF-beta-2 oligonucleotide AP 12009: Results of safety pharmacology and toxicity studies [abstract]. Journal of Cancer Research and Clinical Oncology. 2002;**128**(1):S134

[129] Sierzega M, Jarocki P, Trojan J, et al. Gene immunotherapy of pancreatic cancer using IGF-I antisense approach; preliminary results [Abstract]. Journal of Hepato-Biliary-Pancreatic Surgery. 2002;**9**(1):S226

[130] Trojan J, Kopinski P, Drewa T, et al. Immunogenotherapy of prostate cancer. Urologia Polska. 2003;**56**(2):7-11

[131] Messaoudi S. Recent advances in Hsp90 inhibitors as antitumour agents. Anti-Cancer Agents in Medicinal Chemistry. 2008;**8**:761-782

[132] Goudar RK, Shi Q , Hjelmeland MD, et al. Combination therapy of inhibitors of epidermal growth factor receptor/vascular endothelial growth factor receptor 2 (AEE788) and the mammalian target of rapamycin (RAD001) offers improved glioblastoma tumor growth inhibition. Molecular Cancer Therapy. 2005;**4**:101-112

[133] Lamszus K, Brockman MA, Eckerich C, et al. Inhibition of glioblastoma angiogenesis and invasion by combined treatments directed against vascular endothelial growth factor receptor-2, epidermal growth factor receptor, and vascular endothelial-cadherin. Clinical Cancer Research. 2005;**11**:4934-4940

[134] Reardon DA, Quinn JA, Vredenburgh JJ, et al. Phase 1 trial of gefitinib plus sirolimus in adults with recurrent malignant glioma. Clinical Cancer Research. 2006;**12**:860-868

[135] Halatsch ME, Schmidt U, Behnke-Mursch L, Untenberg A, Wirtz CR. Epidermal growth factor inhibition for the treatment of glioblastoma multiforme and other malignant brain tumours. Cancer Treatment Reviews. 2006;**32**:74-89

[136] Wen PY, Yung WK, Lamborn KR, et al. Phase I/II study of imatinib mesylate for recurrent malignant gliomas: Norty American Brain Tumour Consortium Study 99-08. Clinical Cancer Research. 2006;**12**:4899-4907

[137] Pan Q , Luo X, Chegini N. Blocking neuropilin-1 function has an additive effect with anti-VEGF to inhibit tumor growth. Cancer Cell. 2007;**11**(1):53-67

[138] Trojan LA, Ly A, Upegui-Gonzalez LC, et al. Antisense anti IGF-I therapy of primary hepatic cancer. Journal Africain du Cancer. 2009;**1**:1-10

[139] Biroccio A, Leonett C, Zupi G. The future of antisense therapy: Combination with anticancer treatment. Oncogene. 2003;**22**:6579-6588

[140] Meng Y, Carpentier AF, Chen L, et al. Successful combination of local CpG-ODN and radiotherapy in malignant glioma. International Journal of Cancer. 2005;**116**:992-997

[141] Gonzalez J, Gilbert MR. Treatment of astrocytomas. Current Opinion in Neurology. 2005;**18**:632-638

[142] Jane EP, Premkumar DR, Pollack IF. Coadministration of sorafenib with rottlerin potently inhibits cell proliferation and migration in human malignant glioma cells. Journal of Pharmacology and Experimental Therapy. 2006;**319**:1070-1080

[143] Vega EA, Graner MW, Sampson JH. Combating immunosuppression in glioma. Future Oncology. 2008;**4**(3):433-442

[144] Trojan J. Brain - From Development to Neoplasia and Gene Therapy Solution. Germany: Lambert Academic Publishers; 2018. 150p. ISBN: 978-620-2-08024-8

[145] Dietrich PY, Dutoit V, Tran Thang NN, et al. T cell immunotherapy for malignant glioma: Toward a combined approach. Current Opinion in Oncology. 2010;**22**(6):604-610

[146] Wikipedia—Gene Therapy, History 1990s–2010s

[147] Trojan A, Aristizabal B, Jay LM, et al. Testing of IGF-I biomarker in an ethical context. Advances in Modern Oncology Research. 2016;**2**(4). DOI: 10.18282/amor:v2:i4.58

Chapter 5

Applications of Lipidic and Polymeric Nanoparticles for siRNA Delivery

Behiye Şenel and Gülay Büyükköroğlu

Abstract

The antisense technology that emerged with the discovery of RNA interference nearly 20 years ago has gained a significant place in gene therapy. siRNA, one of two important components of RNA interference, efficiently downregulates gene expression in human cells, so it has the potential to eradicate disease. siRNA delivery systems, which can be applied both systemically and locally in different diseases, have gained significant importance. Naked small RNAs can be delivered directly to cells, but because of their instability, exposure to enzyme degradation, and difficulties in reaching/entering the target cell or tissue in blood stream, these initiatives are failing. For this reason, the method of delivery or encapsulation of siRNA is usually required. Various nanoparticles, nanocapsules, emulsions, micelle systems, metal ion nanoparticles, and nanoconjugates have been used for siRNA delivery. In these transport systems, lipidic and polymeric systems are very attractive due to their advantages such as being biodegradable and biocompatible, safety, being able to electrostatically bind to RNA, long-term stability, well-illuminated structure and features, simple and easy production, etc. Issues such as particle size, zeta potential, and stability of siRNA-loaded system should be taken into consideration in the development of siRNA delivery systems.

Keywords: lipidic nanoparticles, polymeric nanoparticles, nanocarrier, transfection, barriers, siRNA delivery

1. Introduction

Noncoding RNAs have many functions such as gene silencing, DNA imprinting, and demethylation. An increased number of noncoding RNAs have been discovered in gene regulation and RNA processing. Of these, small interfering ribonucleic acid (siRNA) and microRNAs (miRNAs) that can interfere with the translation of the target mRNA transcript are small ncRNAs that are the cleavage products of the dsRNA. MicroRNAs are a class of endogenous RNA that results in mRNA translation inhibition or degradation, which regulates cell differentiation, proliferation, and survival, while synthetic siRNA can initiate the silencing of target genes without interrupting natural mRNA pathways.

siRNA is a promising therapeutic solution preventing gene overexpression in various pathological conditions such as infectious or ocular disease, cancer, and genetic or metabolic disorders. These therapeutic methods are currently being a phenomenon in cancer therapy because siRNA is used to suppress oncogenes and to remove mutations and to illuminate key molecules in the cellular pathways of cancer [1, 2].

It is also effective in personalized gene therapy for several diseases, due to its specificity, compatibility, and targeting ability. Following this strategic discovery, many synthetic siRNAs are designed with the desired sequences to explicitly inhibit any target gene expression [3, 4]. However, naked siRNA is unstable in the bloodstream and cannot effectively pass the cell membranes as well as being immunogenic [5].

There is a need for delivery systems in order to overcome the obstacles and to increase their potentials in the process of transporting siRNAs to the desired destination with minimal adverse effects and safe transportation to target areas. These carriers are usually provided with viral (retrovirus, lentivirus, adenovirus, adeno-associated virus (AAV), cough viruses, human foamy viruses, and baculovirus) and non-viral vectors. Viral vectors are effective tools for transfection vectors which are efficient delivery systems that utilize genetically modified viruses, offering advantages such as continuous gene silencing and the ease of expression of a large number of RNA interference (RNAi) molecules from a transcript [6, 7].

However, safety concerns such as oncogenicity, immunogenicity, viral genome insertion into host chromosomes, and expensive production limit the widespread use of viral vectors [8].

Until now, only one virus-mediated transport system has been authorized for marketing. Glybera® (alipogene tiparvovec using an adeno-associated virus as vector) was the first drug approved by the European Commission in late 2012 to treat lipoprotein lipase deficiency (LPLD). However, in early 2018, the most expensive drug in the world has been withdrawn from the market for financial reasons [9]. Therefore, it is important to design non-viral transport vectors for the in vivo delivery of siRNAs.

These delivery systems are mostly intended to make the siRNA more efficient for interaction with angiogenesis, metastasis, chemoresistance of tumors, and proliferation of cancer cells. Although these systems show encouraging results for possible therapeutic success, many obstacles still exist to implement them in humans, practically.

Delivery systems should not be immunogenic and should not cause undesirable side effects. In normal cells, siRNAs should avoid off-target silencing of genes [10].

The carrier systems should not be defined as foreign particles by the immune system elements, i.e., interferons and cytokines, and should not be eliminated before they reach the target. These difficulties have been overcome by the precise design of the siRNA to the target or by chemical modification of the relevant siRNA molecule.

For this reason, the use of lipidic/polymeric nanoparticles is the most common choice to overcome the above difficulties. These developed nanoparticles can protect the siRNA from plasmatic nucleases and unwanted immune responses, thereby facilitating endocytosis, designed to resist renal clearance; providing low cytotoxicity, stable serum stability, and high structural and functional reliability; delivering the unstable naked siRNA to targeted tumor sites; and reducing interactions with nontarget cells [7].

They can also be used for on-target delivery by adding target-specific ligands to their surface. The most preferred among these transport systems are lipid-based and polymer-based systems. Several technologies and nanoparticle modifications developed in recent years and new nanoparticle raw materials have accelerated the development of siRNA-loaded nanoparticles with the desired structural and functional properties.

DRUG name	Disease or condition	Target	Delivery vector	Phase	Trial number	Company	Recruitment status
CALAA-01	Solid tumors	RRM2	CD/polymer	1	NCT00689065	Calando Pharmaceuticals	Terminated 2008–2013
ALN-VSP02	Solid tumors	KSP, VEGF	LNP	1	NCT00882180	Alnylam Pharmaceuticals	Completed 2009–2011
Atu027	Advanced solid tumors	PKN3	LNP	1	NCT00938574	Silence Therapeutics GmbH	Completed 2009–2013
PRO-040201	Hypercholesterolemia	ApoB	SNALP	1	NCT00927459	Arbutus Biopharma Corporation	Terminated 2009–2010
TKM-080301	Primary or secondary liver cancer	PLK1	LNP	1	NCT01437007	National Cancer Institute (NCI)	Completed 2011–2018
DCR-MYC	Hepatocellular carcinoma	MYC	LNP	1b/2	NCT02314052	Dicerna Pharmaceuticals, Inc.	Terminated 2014–2018
	Solid tumors, multiple myeloma, lymphoma	MYC	LNP	1	NCT02110563	Dicerna Pharmaceuticals, Inc.	Terminated 2014–2017
siRNA-EphA2-DOPC	Advanced solid tumors	EphA2	NL	1	NCT01591356	M.D. Anderson Cancer Center	Recruiting 2012–2018
ND-L02-s0201	Moderate to extensive hepatic fibrosis	HSP47	LNP	1	NCT01858935	Bristol-Myers Squibb	Completed 2014–2017

KSP, kinesin spindle protein; VEGF, vascular endothelial growth factor; PEI, polyethylenimine; NP, neutral liposome; CD, cyclodextrin; PKN3, protein kinase N3; PLK1, polo-like kinase-1; ApoB, MYC oncogene, apolipoprotein B; SNALP, stable nucleic acid lipid particle.

Table 1.
siRNA-based clinical trials using lipidic and polymeric vectors for cancer therapy [12, 13].

Taking advantage of these excellent properties of nanoparticles, various delivery systems for siRNA have recently used the clinical trial phase, and these methods are followed as a very effective and promising treatment for various disease.

As the latest development in this issues, the US Food and Drug Administration approved the Onpattro (patisiran) infusion on 10 August 2018 for the treatment of peripheral nerve disease (polyneuropathy) caused by hereditary transthyretin-mediated amyloidosis (hATTR) in adult patients. It is also the first FDA approval of a new class of drugs called small interfering ribonucleic acid (siRNA) treatment. FDA anticipates that this is the beginning of a new and exciting generation of therapeutics [11].

Patisiran is covered in a lipid nanoparticle (LNP) that carries the drug to the liver, but this carrier molecule can trigger its own immune response. Therefore, steroid, acetaminophen, and antihistamines should be used to reduce the likelihood of immune reaction in patients before taking patisiran administered by intravenous (IV) infusion. Further research is underway to design a drug delivery system that can reach the target tissue without causing an immune response. **Table 1** presents examples of clinical trials and current status of siRNAs prepared with lipidic and polymeric nanoparticle.

2. Physiological barriers for siRNA

The site of action of the SiRNA therapeutics is cytosol. The obstacles to siRNA administration vary depending on the targeted organs, disease, and routes of administration. In general, siRNA therapeutics are preferred as local or systemic injection. The local transport of siRNA has less obstruction compared to systemic administration. The first of the unique features of the local administration is the need to an easy formulation that requires easier production and application and secondly provides application of lower doses that limit intracellular (time-concentration-dependent) immune responses [14].

Therefore, the application is limited to easily accessible tissues such as the skin, eye, or mucosa, but successful results have been achieved. However, for the local administration of siRNA, the nervous system, lung, digestive, vagina, and inner coronary walls were selected as target regions [15].

For example, intranasal inhalation of the siRNA against the respiratory syncytial virus was carried out with TransIT-TKO commercial transfection agent and was found significantly effective in reducing viral infection [16].

In a recent study by Wu and colleagues, they developed novel PEGylated lipoplex-entrapped alginate scaffold system for vaginal epithelium-targeted siRNAs for the treatment of HIV virus infections. They indicated in the study the potential of the biodegradable PLAS system for the sustained delivery of siRNA/oligonucleotides to vaginal epithelium [17].

The main advantage of the systemic method is rapid action and biodistribution but also a wide range of applications. In addition, intravenous or intraperitoneal (IP) injection therapy is successfully applied for many diseases in the clinic. However, it causes significant difficulties for siRNA in systemic transmission. The transition steps of the siRNA from the application site to the target action site are shown in **Figure 1**.

As described above, after intravenous injection (1), siRNA is distributed to organs through the blood stream (3) and also undergoes elimination [7].

The siRNA molecules have unwanted physicochemical properties due to their negative charge, large molecular weight, size, and instability. After systemic administration, the naked siRNA administered without vectors is rapidly degraded by serum endonucleases (4), excreted by the kidney (7), or taken up by the macrophages (APC cells) (5) of the mononuclear phagocyte system (MPS) [7, 18].

The result is a short plasma half-life below <10 minutes, so it cannot have enough time to reach the target and/or perform its functions, and therefore the gene silencing is ineffective. These problems are partially addressed by chemical modifications of the RNA backbone and by the use of nano-sized carriers (2) [7, 60].

Nanoparticle studies showed that the nanoparticles below 6 nm were rapidly excreted by renal excretion and nanoparticles in the range of 150–300 nm were taken by the cells of the MPS in the liver and spleen. It is stated that nanoparticles between 30 and 150 nm can hold in the bone marrow, kidney, etc. In addition, it has been reported that red blood cells (RBCs) affect the transport and distribution of microparticles in human microvasculature (diameter <100). In fact, due to collisions with RBCs, microparticles are pushed toward the artery wall where RBCs are virtually absent depending on the shape and size by a radial movement called the "waterfall effect." This event is also called margination, and they have stated that the extravasation cannot occur unless vectors are exposed to margination [14].

In a study done by D'Apolito et al. [20], they found that 3-μm particles had better marginalization than 1 μm. For this reason, it is seen that the size of the prepared particles could be very effective especially in in vivo experiments.

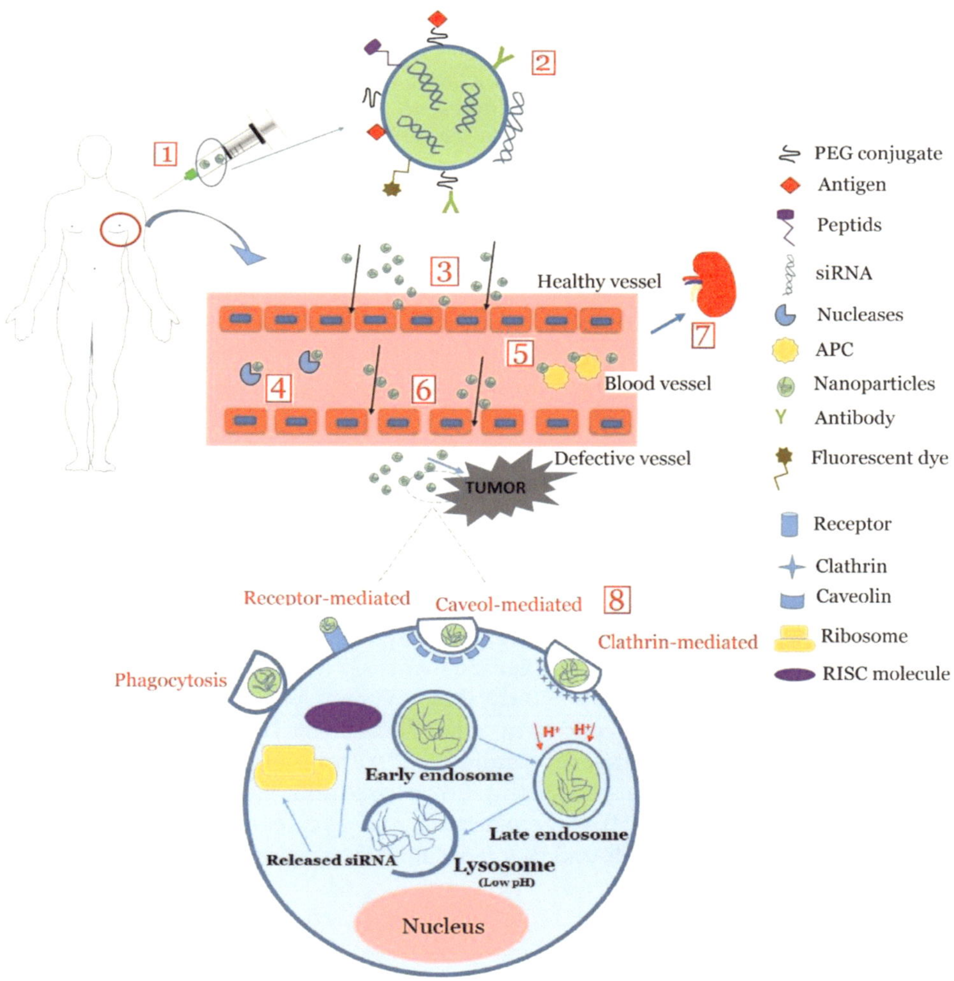

Figure 1.
An illustration of a nanocarrier, barriers at systemic circulatory, mechanisms of uptake of siRNA from cell (modified from the 26th literature). In the following text, the numbers in the figure are mentioned.

The vectors carrying siRNA enter the tissue interstitium following extravasation. After entering the tissue interstitium, siRNA is moved to the target cells across the interstitial space. Transport along the vessel walls can occur via diffusion, convection through the capillary pores, and transcytosis. The diffusion is directed by the concentration gradient.

One of the unique properties of tumor microvessels is leakage (6) from endothelial discontinuity. The pore size of tumor microvessels ranges from 100 to 780 nm in diameter. In contrast, microvessels in most normal tissues have less leakage. For example; the tight junctions between endothelial cells are generally <2 nm, and the pore size in the capillary venules is <6 nm, the endothelium of the renal glomeruli is 40–60 nm, and the sinusoidal endothelium in the liver and spleen has large pore sizes of about 150 nm [19].

Leakage in tumor vessels increases siRNA/carrier extravasation, since the naked siRNA cannot enter the direct cell membrane due to its high molecular weight, large size, and negatively charged phosphate skeleton from the anionic cell membrane; the carrier systems are gaining importance here, again [21, 22].

There is an evidence that endocytosis (8) plays an important role, although not all of the entry mechanisms are well understood. The most common endocytosis used by nanocarriers is clathrin-mediated endocytosis through endocytic route receptor [23].

Rejman et al. [24] showed that the size and nature of the carrier vector affect the internalization mechanism. Nanoparticles of about 1 μm size are taken up via macropinocytosis, and ~120 nm size are taken up via clathrin-mediated endocytosis, whereas nanoparticles ~90 nm are taken up via clathrin/caveolae-independent endocytosis and caveolin-mediated endocytosis [25, 26].

Besides surface properties and size of the nanoparticles, surface modifications of the nanoparticles are also important in siRNA transport. The most important of these surface modifications is the coating of nanoparticles with PEG. The PEGylation is performed to keep the particles in the systemic circulation longer, and the positive results were obtained from until today. However, in addition to this positive effect, it has been reported that the increased PEGylation from 1–2 to 5% mol reduced the transfection efficiency by neutralizing the positive surface load required for siRNA involvement instead of increasing the transfection [27].

After reaching the target cell, the siRNA is subjected to endocytosis internalization, a process involving encapsulated siRNA in endocytic vesicles fused with endosomes. Endocytotic vesicles are initially associated with early endosomes and then mature late endosomes before fusion with lysosomes in the cell. Lysosomes are then formed. After internalization into the cell, the siRNA should escape from the fragmentation in the endosomes and be released from the carrier to the cytosol in order to be loaded to RNA-induced silencing complex (RISC) [28].

Sardo et al. found that endosomal escape increased with another modification with pH-sensitive polymers. In this study, they prepared a siRNA delivery system based on inulin (Inu), a plenty and natural polysaccharide. Inu was functionalized via the conjugation with diethylenetriamine (DETA) residues to form the complex Inu-DETA. The results of the study showed that while homogenous diffusion of siRNA was performed in JHH6 cytoplasm via micropinocytosis and clathrin-mediated endocytosis, it was found that it did not allow caveola-mediated passage and no siRNA activity [29].

3. Types of nanoparticulate delivery systems for siRNA delivery

This section focuses on the biodegradable non-viral lipids and polymeric nanosystems used in the transport of synthetic siRNA. These nanoparticles used as drug delivery vehicles are carriers having a particle size of <100 nm. They are composed of different biodegradable materials, such as natural or synthetic polymers, lipids, or metal.

The main advantages of nanoparticles used as drug carriers are achieving appropriate particle size, using of physiological lipids (e.g., triglycerides) and organic polymers (e.g., chitosan) to reduce immunogenicity, stimulating interferon-γ production and natural killer (NK) cells, activating antitumor immunity to increase the effectiveness of treatment, prolongation of blood circulation in blood, and feasibility of variable routes of administration; they can be viewed and monitored by marking.

However, they have some disadvantages; for example, the substances used during the formulation and the preparation methods may cause the increase of toxicity, sometimes failing to carry the siRNA into the cell or insufficient accumulation at the target site, and problems in the stability of lipidic structures like liposomes. These limitations, however, can be overcome by selecting the appropriate lipid or polymers. The advantages thus outweigh the disadvantages [30].

3.1 Lipid-based nanoparticle delivery systems

Lipid-based siRNA delivery systems include liposomes, micelles, microemulsions, ionizable lipids and lipid nanoparticles, and solid lipid nanoparticles.

3.1.1 Liposomes

Liposomes are spherical vesicles consisting of an aqueous core together with a bilayer phospholipid structure which contain natural body components (e.g., lipids, sterols) and are biologically compatible and biodegradable. Furthermore, liposomes are popular siRNA carriers due to their relative simplicity and well-known pharmaceutical properties. The amphipathic nature of liposomes allows the use of a wide range of hydrophilic and hydrophobic drugs. The hydrophilic molecules show a greater affinity between the hydrophilic head groups of the phospholipid bilayer and the aqueous core of the liposomes, while the hydrophobic molecules intercalate between the fatty acyl chains of the two lipid layers [31].

As analogues of biological membranes, liposomes are fused with the plasma membrane and are processed by endocytosis, and the genetic material is released into the cytoplasm. Cationic liposomes form complexes with negatively charged anionic siRNAs and polycations, and the complex is called as a "lipoplex."

However, due to their positive charge, cationic liposomes can lead to dose-dependent cytotoxicity and inflammatory response, and the complexes can interact nonspecifically with negatively charged serum proteins. In order to solve these problems, successful tests were taken in preclinical studies of EphA2-targeted siRNA therapeutic using neutral lipids such as 1,2-dioleoyl-sn-glycero-3-phosphatidylcholine (DOPC), which proved to effectively reduce cellular toxicity [31].

Several strategies have been implemented to overcome the disadvantages of existing lipid-based systems. Modification of the lipid structure or formulation methods can reduce toxicity and improve transfection. The inclusion of fusogenic lipids, such as dioleoylphosphatidylethanolamine (DOPE), or the use of a cationic lipid consisting of biodegradable ester bonds such as DOTAP may retain toxic effects at a relatively short or moderate level and also may increase the endosomal release of siRNA [32].

3.1.2 Solid lipid nanoparticles

SLNs having a size range of 50–1000 nm were composed from various lipids which are solid form at body or room temperature and can be stabilized with surfactant or surfactant mixture. SLNs consist of a lipid core surrounded by a surfactant layer in an aqueous dispersion [33].

While being among the most effective carriers for both hydrophilic and hydrophobic drugs, such as liposomes, the solid, lipophilic nucleus of SLNs may have difficulty carrying RNA molecules that are hydrophilic and polyanionic. Therefore, it can be used successfully for gene delivery by addition of cationic lipids to SLNs which provide a positive surface potential [34].

SLNs can be easily prepared by various methods such as hot or cold homogenization, sonication, solvent evaporation, etc., and also they have high physical stability and low cytotoxicity [35].

Studies with siRNAs that have been adsorbed or encapsulated into SLNs have also shown positive results in the literature. For example, Şenel et al. [36] pointed out that Bcl-2-targeted siRNAs encapsulated into SLNs prepared by sonication method showed an activity to be able to compete with Lipofectamine in the liposomal form commercially used.

3.1.3 Nanostructured lipid carriers (NLCs)

Nanostructured lipid carriers (NLCs) are new second-generation lipid carriers that combine the advantages of different nanocarriers. These are solid lipid-core-modified SLNs in which the lipid phase may comprise solid or liquid forms at ambient temperature [37].

Compared to SLNs, NLCs have greater loading capacity and less water in the dispersion, making them more stable for storage. There was no difference in biotoxicity. Studies have shown that NLCs can be used as a new delivery tool for the genetic treatment of disease. Taratula et al. prepared a multifunctional NLC system containing two siRNAs against cellular resistance to doxorubicin or paclitaxel targeting lung cancer cells. It has been found that the system successfully increases the antitumor activity of the anticancer drug [38, 39].

NLCs can also be modified to achieve targeting and sustained release. For example, by manipulating the degradation times of NLCs, it has made possible to obtain long-acting siRNAs. This design raised the continuous release of siRNAs to 9 days (with a A-tailored nanostructure carrier design delivering survivin-siRNA); this also facilitates clinical practice of siRNA treatment [40].

3.1.4 Ionizable lipids and lipid nanoparticles (LNPs)

Recently, new lipid types have been proposed to the delivery of RNA interference molecules. Advanced LNP siRNA systems are lipid-based particles with diameters <100 nm. These may consist of a mixture of an ionizable amino lipid (e.g., heptatriaconta-6,9,28,31-tetraen-19-yl-4-(dimethylamino)butanoate, DLin-MC3-DMA), a phosphatidylcholine, cholesterol, and a coat lipid (polyethylene glycol-dimiris glycerol) in a 50:10:38.5:1.5 molar ratio [41].

These lipids developed for the encapsulation of negatively charged genetic materials exhibit pH-dependent charge change. These lipids are positive at acidic pH and are neutral at physiological pH. Thus, under acidic conditions, nucleic acids are encapsulated in the nanoparticle and have a minimum positive charge density in the bloodstream. LNP siRNA systems are produced by rapidly mixing the lipids in ethanol with the siRNA in aqueous buffer (pH 4.0) followed by removal of ethanol via dialysis against PBS buffer after the pH is raised to 7.4 [42].

The genetic material carrier formulations generated by ionizable cationic lipids have been shown to be of significant success in in vivo activity after the initial administration in hepatocytes. Other tissues used for gene silencing include macrophages, osteoclasts, and osteoblasts in the "hard" bone and distal tumor cells [43, 44].

Other siRNA administration methods have used lipid-like molecules called "lipidoids" for the delivery of siRNA. Lipidoid delivery systems are similar to ionizable cationic LNP systems due to the use of lipid-like molecules, cholesterol, and PEG-lipid. The most important difference of LNPs using lipidoid is that the lipidoid molecules have an extra positive charge because they have a large number of protonizable amine bound to various acyl chains. Similar to studies with cationic lipids, lipidoid systems developed by screening programs have been described in the literature [45].

Ball et al. developed a potent and nontoxic lipidoid nanoparticle (LNP) for intestinal epithelial cells. In the initial studies, it was reported that GAPDH siRNA-loaded LNPs for Caco-2 cells mediated strong, dose-dependent, and resistant gene silencing with a single 10-nM dose for 1 week [46].

3.2 Polymer-based delivery

Polymers of natural and synthetic origin have been used for various biomedical applications including drug targeting, imaging, gene therapy, prostheses, tissue engineering, etc. Because of their reproducible properties in terms of molecular weight, degradation, and mechanical properties, synthetic polymers are attractive for therapeutic applications. The most commonly used polymers include polyethylenimine (PEI), PLGA, PEG, PLL, PLA, etc. However, the synthetic polymers have the disadvantage biologically, such as they can turn into undesirable side effects or fail to achieve the desired bioactivity and biocompatibility. On the other hand, natural polymers are abundant and are similar to components of those found in biological extracellular matrices. Thus, the natural polymers have high bioactivity and biocompatibility. Natural polymers include polysaccharides, proteins, and polyesters [47].

3.2.1 Synthetic polymers

Linear or branched cationic polymers are effective transfection agents for genetic material. The structural and chemical properties of these polymers are well known. This makes them advantageous for siRNA transport. The positively charged polymers form "polyplexes" with negatively charged nucleic acid phosphates through electrostatic interactions [48].

The polymer size, the molecular weight, the degree of polymer branching, and the charge density, as well as the composition of the formulation medium and the positive and negative charges ratio between of the polymer and the oligonucleotides, affect the transfection efficiency and biological activity of the polyplexes.

Synthetic-based cationic polymers such as PLL, PLA, and PEI are the most studied polymers for in vitro and in vivo transport of siRNA. The size of the complexes is one of the most important factors affecting cellular uptake. Due to their small size, the cationic polymers generally complex with the genetic material more effectively than lipids. In addition, owing to being mostly synthetic, they have some special feature such as customized size, branching, and composition, and these features can be easily changed [49].

These polymers used for siRNA delivery is well-studied, biodegradable, biocompatible, and capable of exhibiting nucleic acid sustained release in pharmaceutical applications for decades.

PEI was used to create cationic charges on the surface of PLGA particles, which allowed the complexation of nucleic acids on the surface of the particles [50].

In a study done by Patil and Panyam [51], siRNA encapsulation studies were performed in PLGA nanoparticles. These nanoparticles were prepared by the solvent evaporation method. In this method, a cationic polymer, PEI, was added to the PLGA matrix, and ultimately it has been reported that nanoparticles can penetrate into the cell at twice the rate.

Furthermore, cationic polymers with high charge densities have "proton sponge" properties that stimulate escape from endosomes and protect genetic materials from degradation. For example, PEI, by pulling and sustaining a significant amount of protons, induces osmotic swelling and rupture of endosomes, causing the genetic material to be released from the nanoparticles in the cytoplasm and thus preventing the transport to lysosomes and degradation of genetic material [52].

In another study, the hydrogel scaffold based on polyamidoamine (PAMAM) dendrimer cross-linked with dextran aldehyde was prepared to improve the stability of the nanoparticle. These nanoparticle systems were found to be effective for gene silencing [53].

3.2.2 Natural polymers

Many polysaccharides in natural polymer structure are used for siRNA. Polysaccharides are generally biocompatible polymers. The main advantage is the presence of different functional groups (i.e., carboxyl, hydroxyl, amine) which enable functionalization to obtain structural heterogeneity and copolymers [54].

The most commonly used polysaccharides for siRNA administration include chitosan, which contains both biodegradable, biocompatible, low-cost, low cytotoxicity hydroxyl and amines. The presence of primary amino groups (pKa $\approx$ 6) makes the chitosan a polycation that promotes the association with nucleic acids and also the formation of polyplex [55].

In order to increase the solubility of chitosan, various modifications have been done and water-soluble chitololigosaccharides have been obtained. These chitololigosaccharides were used for delivery of the siRNA [35, 56].

Collagen is another biologically compatible and safe natural polymer and is a suitable carrier for drug delivery. In a study performed by Peng et al., localized and sustained release of siRNA-loaded collagen formulations were prepared for use in vivo gastric cancer, and positive results were obtained [57].

3.3 Lipid-polymer hybrid nanoparticles

Lipid-polymer hybrid nanoparticles (LPNs) were developed to eliminate the disadvantages of polymeric and lipid-based nanoparticles. The precious properties of LPNs containing polymer cores and lipid shells carry the complementary properties of both materials. In a study on the administration of LPNs in cancer treatment, the lipid/rPAA-Chol polymer hybrid nanoparticles were modified with PEG and T7 peptide; tumor has been shown to be largely inhibited without activating the immune system [58].

In another study, LPNs were used for the antitumoral effect in the pancreatic tumor model in combination with hypoxia-inducible factor 1α (HIF1alpha)-targeted siRNA and gemitabicin. This prepared LPN complex showed an excellent ability to inhibit tumor metastasis in an orthotopic tumor model [59].

4. Conclusion

In recent years, siRNA has been widely used as a promising therapeutic phenomenon to many pathological conditions. Progress has been made in researching target genes and in the development of delivery systems for siRNA. However, challenges remain for successful clinical application of RNAi-based therapeutics. Safety concerns are the main reason for the withdrawal of clinical trials of some RNAi therapies.

Since its discovery, siRNA therapeutics have been actively used because of their high specificity, easy modifications, and unlimited therapeutic targets. However, the instability in the bloodstream and the problems with the accumulation in the target region necessitated the application of these therapeutics in a transport system.

The lipidic and polymeric nanoparticle systems described in this chapter are one step ahead the systems than other nanoparticle systems and have been proven to be of importance in these delivery processes in recent years. New modified systems are being developed to ensure safe and targeted distribution of siRNA. According to the results obtained from studies, new formulations are expected to reach clinical trials very soon such as patisiran.

Conflict of interest

The authors report no conflicts of interest. The authors alone are responsible for the content of and writing of this article.

Author details

Behiye Şenel* and Gülay Büyükköroğlu
Faculty of Pharmacy, Anadolu University, Eskisehir, Turkey

*Address all correspondence to: behiyek@anadolu.edu.tr

IntechOpen

© 2019 The Author(s). Licensee IntechOpen. This chapter is distributed under the terms of the Creative Commons Attribution License (http://creativecommons.org/licenses/by/3.0), which permits unrestricted use, distribution, and reproduction in any medium, provided the original work is properly cited.

References

[1] Van de Veire S, Stalmans I, Heindryckx F, Oura H, Tijeras-Raballand A, Schmidt T, et al. Pharmacological and genetic evidence for the efficacy of PlGF inhibition in cancer and eye disease. Cell. 2010;**141**:178-190. DOI: 10.1016/j.cell.2010.02.039

[2] Zhao M, Sun J, Zhao Z. Synergetic regulatory networks mediated by oncogene-driven microRNAs and transcription factors in serous ovarian cancer. Molecular BioSystems. 2013;**9**:3187-3198. DOI: 10.1039/c3mb70172g

[3] Fellmann C, Lowe SW. Stable RNA interference rules for silencing. Nature Cell Biology. 2014;**16**:10-18. DOI: 10.1038/ncb2895

[4] Lee SJ, Kim MJ, Kwon IC, Roberts TM. Delivery strategies and potential targets for siRNA in major cancer types. Advanced Drug Delivery Reviews. 2015;**104**:2-15. DOI: 10.101/j.addr.2016.05.010

[5] Wang J, Mi P, Lin G, Wáng YXJ, Liu G, Chen X. Imaging-guided delivery of RNAi for anticancer treatment. Advanced Drug Delivery Reviews. 2015;**104**:44-60. DOI: 10.1016/j.addr.2016.01.008

[6] Grimm D. Small silencing RNAs: State-of-the-art. Advanced Drug Delivery Reviews. 2009;**61**(9):672-703. DOI: 10.1016/j.addr.2009.05.002

[7] David S, Pitard B, Benoît JP, Passirani C. Non-viral nanosystems for systemic siRNA delivery. Pharmacological Research. 2010;**62**(2):100-114. DOI: 10.1016/j.phrs.2009.11.013

[8] Giacca M, Zacchigna S. Virus-mediated gene delivery for human gene therapy. Journal of Controlled Release. 2012;**161**(2):377-388. DOI: 10.1016/j.jconrel.2012.04.008

[9] Glybera: EPAR-Product Information [Internet]. 2017. Available from: https://www.ema.europa.eu/documents/product-information/glybera-epar-product-information_en.pdf [Accessed: 30 September 2018]

[10] Jackson AL, Burchard J, Schelter J, Chau BN, Cleary M, Lim L, et al. Widespread siRNA "off-target" transcript silencing mediated by seed region sequence complementarity. RNA. 2006;**12**:1179-1187. DOI: 10.1261/rna.25706

[11] FDA approves first-of-its kind targeted RNA-based therapy to treat a rare disease [Internet]. 2018. Available from: https://www.fda.gov/NewsEvents/Newsroom/PressAnnouncements/ucm616518.htm [Accessed: 30 September 2018]

[12] Clinical Trials [Internet]. 2018. Available from: https://clinicaltrials.gov [Accessed: 30 September 2018

[13] Chen X, Mangala LS, Rodriguez-Aguayo C, Kong X, Lopez-Berestein G, Sood AK. RNA interference-based therapy and its delivery systems. Cancer Metastasis Reviews. 2018;**37**(1):107-124. DOI: 10.1007/s10555-017-9717-6

[14] Barba AA, Cascone S, Caccavo D, Lamberti G, Chiarappa G, Abrami M, et al. Engineering approaches in siRNA delivery. International Journal of Pharmaceutics. 2017;**525**(2):343-358. DOI: 10.1016/j.ijpharm.2017.02.032

[15] Vicentini FT, Borgheti-Cardoso LN, Depieri LV, de Macedo Mano D, Abelha TF, Petrilli R, et al. Delivery systems and local administration routes for therapeutic siRNA. Pharmaceutical Research. 2013;**30**:915-931. DOI: 10.1007/s11095-013-0971-1

[16] Bitko V, Musiyenko A, Shulyayeva O, Barik S. Inhibition of respiratory viruses by nasally administered siRNA. Nature Medicine. 2005;**11**(1):50-55. DOI: 10.1038/nm1164

[17] Wu SY, Chang HI, Burgess M, McMillan NA. Vaginal delivery of siRNA using a novel PEGylated lipoplex-entrapped alginate scaffold system. Journal of Controlled Release. 2011;**155**(3):418-426. DOI: 10.1016/j.jconrel.2011.02.002

[18] Van de Water FM, Boerman OC, Wouterse AC, Peters JG, Russel FG, Masereeuw R. Intravenously administered short interfering RNA accumulates in the kidney and selectively suppresses gene function in renal proximal tubules. Drug Metabolism and Disposition. 2006;**34**(8):1393-1397. DOI: 10.1124/dmd.106.009555

[19] Jain A, Jain A, Gulbake A, Hurkat P, Jain SK. Solid Tumors: A Review. International Journal of Pharmacy and Pharmaceutical Sciences. 2011;**3**(5):45-51

[20] D'Apolito R, Tomaiuolo G, Taraballi F, Minardi S, Kirui D, Liu X, et al. Red blood cells affect the margination of microparticles in synthetic microcapillaries and intravital microcirculation as a function of their size and shape. Journal of Controlled Release. 2015;**217**:263-272. DOI: 10.1016/j.jconrel.2015.09.013

[21] Goula D, Becker N, Lemkine GF, Normandie P, Rodrigues J, Mantero S, et al. Rapid crossing of the pulmonary endothelial barrier by polyethylenimine/DNA complexes. Gene Therapy. 2000;**7**(6):499-504. DOI: 10.1038/sj.gt.3301113

[22] Wullner U, Neef I, Tur MK, Barth S. Targeted delivery of short interfering RNAs—Strategies for in vivo delivery. Recent Patents on Anti-Cancer Drug Discovery. 2009;**4**:1-8. DOI: 10.2174/157489209787002506

[23] Palakurthi S, Yellepeddi VK, Kumar A. Nanocarriers for cytosolic drug and gene delivery in cancer therapy. In: Anna M, Olsztynska S, editors. Biomedical Engineering, Trends, Research and Technologies. Croatia: InTech; 2011. pp. 245-272. DOI: 10.5772/12918

[24] Rejman J, Oberle V, Zuhorn IS, Hoekstra D. Size-dependent internalization of particles via the pathways of clathrin- and caveolae-mediated endocytosis. The Biochemical Journal. 2004;**377**:159-169. DOI: 10.1042/BJ20031253

[25] Petros RA, DeSimone JM. Strategies in the design of nanoparticles for therapeutic applications. Nature Reviews. Drug Discovery. 2010;**9**(8):615-627. DOI: 10.1038/nrd2591

[26] Şenel B, Büyükköroğlu G. Nanocarriers for vaccine and gene delivery application. In: Barkat A, Harshita AB, Beg S, Ahmad FJ, editors. Multifunctional Nanocarriers for Contemporary Healthcare Applications. USA: IGI Global; 2018. pp. 381-414. DOI: 10.4018/978-1-5225-4781-5.ch014

[27] Santel A, Aleku M, Keil O, Endruschat J, Esche V, Fisch G, et al. A novel siRNA-lipoplex technology for RNA interference in the mouse vascular endothelium. Gene Therapy. 2006;**13**(16):1222-1234. DOI: 10.1038/sj.gt.3302777

[28] Mukherjee S, Ghosh RN, Maxfield FR. Endocytosis. Physiological Reviews. 1997;**77**(3):759-803. DOI: 10.1152/physrev.1997.77.3.759

[29] Sardo C, Farra R, Licciardi M, Dapas B, Scialabba C, Giammona G, et al. Development of a simple, biocompatible and cost-effective inulin-diethylenetriamine based siRNA

delivery system. European Journal of Pharmaceutical Sciences. 2015;**75**:60-71. DOI: 10.1016/j.ejps.2015.03.021

[30] Tatiparti K, Sau S, Kashaw SK, Iyer AK. siRNA delivery strategies: A comprehensive review of recent developments. Nanomaterials (Basel). 2017;**7**(4):77. DOI: 10.3390/nano7040077

[31] Wagner MJ, Mitra R, MJ MA, Baze W, Barnhart K, Wu SY, et al. Preclinical mammalian safety studies of EphARNA (DOPC nanoliposomal EphA2-targeted siRNA). Molecular Cancer Therapeutics. 2017;**16**(6):1114-1123. DOI: 10.1158/1535-7163.MCT-16-0541

[32] Dominska M, Dykxhoorn DM. Breaking down the barriers: siRNA delivery and endosome escape. Journal of Cell Science. 2010;**123**:1183-1189. DOI: 10.1242/jcs. 066399

[33] Chauhan H, Mohapatra S, Munt DJ, Chandratre S, Dash A. Physical-chemical characterization and formulation considerations for solid lipid nanoparticles. AAPS PharmSciTech. 2016;**17**(3):640-651. DOI: 10.1208/s12249015-0394-x

[34] Botto C, Mauro N, Amore E, Martorana E, Giammona G, Bondi ML. Surfactant effect on the physicochemical characteristics of cationic solid lipid nanoparticles. International Journal of Pharmaceutics. 2017;**516**(1-2):334-341. DOI: 10. 1016/j.ijpharm.2016.11.052

[35] Mukherjee S, Ray S, Thakur RS. Solid lipid nanoparticles: a modern formulation approach in drug delivery system. Indian Journal of Pharmaceutical Sciences. 2009;**71**(4):349-358. DOI:10.4103/0250-474X.57282

[36] Şenel B, Büyükköroğlu G, Yazan Y. Solid lipid and chitosan particulate systems for delivery of siRNA. Pharmazie. 2015;**8**:698-705. DOI: 10.1691/ph.2015.5026

[37] Kaur S, Nautyal U, Singh R, Singh S, Devi A. Nanostructure lipid carrier (NLC): The new generation of lipid nanoparticles. Asian Pacific Journal of Health Science. 2015;**2**(2):76-93

[38] Han Y, Li Y, Zhang P, Sun J, Li X, Sun X, et al. Nanostructured lipid carriers as novel drug delivery system for lung cancer gene therapy. Pharmaceutical Development and Technology. 2016;**21**(3):277-281. DOI: 10.3109/10837450.2014.996900

[39] Taratula O, Kuzmov A, Shah M, Garbuzenko OB, Minko T. Nanostructured lipid carriers as multifunctional nanomedicine platform for pulmonary co-delivery of anticancer drugs and siRNA. Journal of Controlled Release. 2013;**171**(3):349-357. DOI: 10.1016/j.jconrel.2013.04.018

[40] Xue HY, Wong HL. Tailoring nanostructured solid lipid carriers for time-controlled intracellular siRNA kinetics to sustain RNAi-mediated chemosensitization. Biomaterials. 2011;**32**(10):2662-2672. DOI: 10.1016/j.biomaterials.2010. 12.029

[41] Tam YYC, Chen S, Cullis PR. Advances in lipid nanoparticles for siRNA delivery. Pharmaceutics. 2013;**5**:498507. DOI: 10.3390/pharmaceutics5030498

[42] Basha G, Novobrantseva TI, Rosin N, Tam YY, Hafez IM, Wong MK, et al. Influence of cationic lipid composition on gene silencing properties of lipid nanoparticle formulations of siRNA in antigen-presenting cells. Molecular Therapy. 2011;**19**:2186-2200. DOI: 10.1038/mt.2011.190

[43] Basha G, Ordobadi M, Scott WR, Cottle A, Liu Y, Wang H, et al. Lipid nanoparticle delivery of siRNA to osteocytes leads to effective silencing of

SOST and inhibition of sclerostin in vivo. Molecular Therapy--Nucleic Acids. 2016;**5**:1-15. DOI: 10.1038/mtna.2016.68

[44] Lee JB, Zhang K, Tam YY, Tam YK, Belliveau NM, Sung VY, et al. Lipid nanoparticle siRNA systems for silencing the androgen receptor in human prostate cancer in vivo. International Journal of Cancer. 2012;**131**:781-790. DOI: 10.1002/ijc.27361

[45] Lin PJC, Tam YK, Cullis PR. Development and clinical applications of siRNA-encapsulated lipid nanoparticles in cancer. Journal of Clinical Lipidology. 2014;**9**(3):317-331. DOI: 10.2217/CLP.14.27

[46] Ball RL, Knapp CM, Whitehead KA. Lipidoid nanoparticles for siRNA delivery to the intestinal epithelium: In vitro investigations in a Caco-2 model. PLoS ONE. 2015;**10**:1-12. DOI: 10.1371/journal.pone.0133154

[47] Aravamudhan A, Ramos DM, Nada AA, Kumbar SG. Natural polymers: Polysaccharides and their derivatives for biomedical applications. In: Kumbar SG, Laurencin CT, Deng M, editors. Natural and Synthetic Biomedical Polymers. USA: Elsevier; 2014. pp. 67-89. DOI: 10.1016/B978-0-12-396983-5.00004-1

[48] Rafael D, Andrade F, Arranja A, Luís S, Videira M. Lipoplexes and polyplexes: Gene delivery applications. In: Mishra M, editor. Encyclopedia of Biomedical Polymers and Polymeric Biomaterials. USA: CRC Press Taylor & Francis Group; 2015. pp. 4335-4347. DOI: 10.1081/E-EBPP-120050058

[49] Tros IC, Sun Y, Düzgüneş N. Gene delivery by lipoplexes and polyplexes. European Journal of Pharmaceutical Sciences. 2010;**40**(3):159-170. DOI: 10.1016/j.ejps.2010.03.019

[50] Zhang XQ, Intra J, Salem AK. Comparative study of poly (lactic-co-glycolic acid)-poly ethyleneimine-plasmid DNA microparticles prepared using double emulsion methods. Journal of Microencapsulation. 2008;**25**(1):1-12. DOI: 10.1080/02652040701659347

[51] Patil Y, Panyam J. Polymeric nanoparticles for siRNA delivery and gene silencing. International Journal of Pharmaceutics. 2009;**367**(1-2):195-203. DOI: 10.1016/j.ijpharm.2008.09.039

[52] Wang J, Lu Z, Wientjes MG, Au JLS. Delivery of siRNA Therapeutics: Barriers and Carriers. The AAPS Journal. 2010;**12**(4):492-503. DOI: 10.1208/s12248-010-9210-4

[53] Segovia N, Pont M, Oliva N, Ramos V, Borrós S, Artzi N. Hydrogel doped with nanoparticles for local sustained release of siRNA in breast cancer. Advanced Healthcare Materials. 2015;**4**:271-280. DOI: 10.1002/adhm.201400235

[54] Cavallaro G, Sardo C, Craparo EF, Porsio B, Giammona G. Polymeric nanoparticles for siRNA delivery: Production and applications. International Journal of Pharmaceutics. 2017;**525**(2):313-333. DOI: 10.1016/j.ijpharm.2017.04.008

[55] Ragelle H, Vandermeulen G, Préat V. Chitosan-based siRNA delivery systems. Journal of Controlled Release. 2013;**172**:207-218. DOI: 10.1016/j.jconrel.2013.08.005

[56] Mao S, Sun W, Kissel T. Chitosan-based formulations for delivery of DNA and siRNA. Advanced Drug Delivery Reviews. 2010;**62**(1):12-27. DOI: 10.1016/j.addr.2009.08.004

[57] Peng H, Yang H, Song L, Zhou Z, Sun J, Du Y, et al. Sustained delivery of siRNA/PEI complex from in situ forming hydrogels potently inhibits the proliferation of gastric cancer. Journal of Experimental & Clinical

Cancer Research. 2016;**35**(1):35-57. DOI: 10.1186/s13046-016-0334-y

[58] Gao LY, Liu XY, Chen CJ, Wang JC, Feng Q, Yu MZ, et al. Core-shell type lipid/rPAA-Chol polymer hybrid nanoparticles for in vivo siRNA delivery. Biomaterials. 2014;**35**(6):2066-2078. DOI: 10.1016/j.biomaterials.2013.11.046

[59] Zhao X, Li F, Li Y, Wang H, Ren H, Chen J, et al. Co-delivery of HIF1alpha siRNA and gemcitabine via biocompatible lipid-polymer hybrid nanoparticles for effective treatment of pancreatic cancer. Biomaterials. 2015;**46**:13-25. DOI: org/10.1016/j.biomaterials.2014.12.028

[60] Xu C, Wang J. Delivery systems for siRNA drug development in cancer therapy. Asian Journal of Pharmaceutics. 2015;**10**(1):1-12. DOI: 10.1016/j.ajps.2014.08.011

Chapter 6

Therapeutic Implication of miRNA in Human Disease

Andrew Walayat, Meizi Yang and DaLiao Xiao

Abstract

MicroRNAs (miRNAs) are a class of short non-coding RNA molecules that are involved in development and diseases. Early studies are focusing on the miRNA profile as a biomarker in disease. As discovery of human miRNAs increased in the setting of disease, the research focus was gradually shifted towards miRNA therapeutic strategy for diagnostic and treatment of disease. Increasing evidences suggest that miRNAs are the next important class of antisense therapeutic molecules, which have significant advantage over antisense such as siRNAs because miRNAs are naturally occurring endogenous molecules. Aberrant alteration of the endogenous miRNAs has been linked to the development of certain diseases. Correcting these altered miRNAs by their mimics or inhibitors has been developed as potential therapeutic approaches. Some of the miRNA-based therapeutics are processed in preclinical and clinical trial for treatment hepatitis C, liver cancer, and other diseases. Currently, the major focus in the development of miRNA-based therapeutics is how to increase the miRNA stability and optimize delivery systems for specific disease with minimal off-target effect. This chapter will first overview the miRNA biogenesis, patho- and physiologic function, and regulation of miRNA molecules. Then, we discuss the miRNA-based potential therapeutic approaches and implication in disease.

Keywords: miRNA, function, disease biomarker, therapeutics

1. Introduction

MicroRNAs (miRNAs) belong to a family of small non-protein-coding RNAs with a single strand of 18–25 nucleotides that regulate multiple target genes at the post-transcriptional level. Functionally, miRNAs bind to 6–8 bp seed sequences in the 3' Untranslated Region (3' UTR) of targets mRNA and induce mRNA degradation or repression of protein translation. The term "non-coding RNA" is commonly defined a group of RNA that does not encode a protein. With a rapid advancement of molecular technology, many new classes of noncoding RNA have been founded. Among those noncoding RNAs, miRNA has attracted considerable attention because its endogenous origin and its role in the regulation of gene makes it more likely target for drug discovery and potential biomarker for specific disease.

miRNA research is a relatively new topic, with research ranging back for the past 25 years; it has its beginnings in its detection in *C. elegans* in 1993 and its detection in humans in 2000 [1]. Their use in transgenic mice in 2005 to eventually efficacy studies of modified inhibitors of miRNAs in primates in 2010 illustrates the explosion of research surrounding miRNAs in just 5 years. There are now over 2000 miRNAs that have been discovered in humans and it is believed that they collectively regulate one third of the genes in the genome [2]. miRNAs have been linked to many human diseases and are being pursued as clinical diagnostics and as therapeutic targets, showing promise in many fields, ranging from cancer therapy to cardiac disease, to even suggestions as a potential biomarker for numerous diseases and treatment responses. This chapter will briefly discuss the miRNAs biogenesis, their function, regulation, and implication in disease, then discuss the miRNA-based therapeutic strategies, their therapeutic implication in diseases, and some of the current clinical trials involving miRNAs.

2. miRNA biochemical synthesis

miRNAs are encoded in the genomes (inter or intragenic) and are transcribed from genes located in nuclear DNA; however, such genes are not eventually translated into protein [3]. These transcribed genes are typically longer than the eventual gene product miRNA and undergo much post-transcriptional modification between initial transcription and the functional miRNA end-product. After initial transcription of the DNA sequence, the miRNA sequence contains a reverse-complement base pair segment that forms a double stranded RNA hairpin loop. The entire DNA transcript, including the double stranded RNA loop, constitute the primary miRNA structure (called pri-miRNA). Pri-miRNA is usually several kilobases long and has local stem loop structures. The primary transcripts undergo further processing in the nucleus. The ribonucleases Drosha and DiGeorge syndrome critical region gene 8 (DGCR8) complex are mainly involved in the pri-miRNA processing, which is cleaved at the stem of the hairpin structure and generates a hairpin intermediate of about 70–100 nucleotides, called pre-miRNA.

The pre-miRNA is then transported out of the nucleus to the cytoplasm for further processing to become mature miRNA. There are nuclear pore complexes in the nuclear membrane where the pre-miRNA can be transported out of the nucleus by means of the RanGTP-dependent nuclear transport receptor exportin 5. In the cytoplasm, the pre-miRNA is processed by another ribonuclease, Dicer to create a mature miRNA. The mature miRNA is a double-stranded miRNA of variable length (~18–25 nucleotides). After the generation of mature miRNA duplex by Dicer, the miRNA duplex is incorporated into an Ago family protein complex, which generates an effector complex. Then one strand of the miRNA is degraded, whereas the other strand remains bound to Ago as mature miRNA (guide strand). After strand separation, the guide strand or mature miRNA is incorporated into an RNA-induced silencing complex (RISC). After loading, the miRNA promotes the RISC to its target mRNA and induces mRNA degradation or translational repression (see **Figure 1**).

3. Functions of miRNAs

The general function of miRNA is oriented towards gene silencing [3, 4]. miRNAs specifically recognize mRNA and downregulate gene expression by one of the two post-transcriptional mechanisms: (1) translational repression and (2) mRNA cleavage. The determinant of the regulatory mechanism process is mainly dependent on the degree of

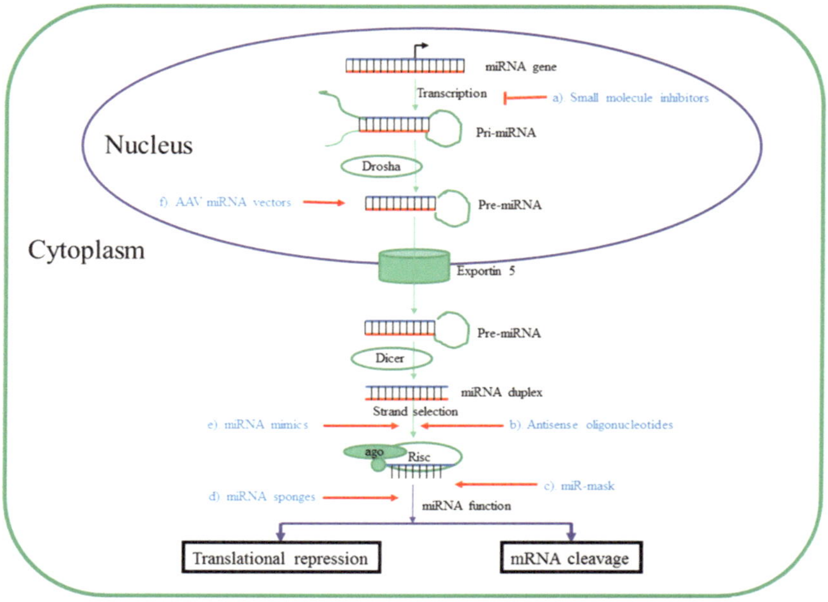

Figure 1.
miRNA biogenesis, function, and strategies for miRNA-based therapies. miRNA is transcribed from miRNA gene via RNA polymerase II as pri-miRNA and cleaved by Drosha complex in the nucleus. The resulting precursor miRNA (pre-miRNA) is exported to the cytoplasm via exportin 5 complex. In the cytoplasm, Dicer complex cleaves pre-miRNA to form mature miRNA duplex. The strand is separated and the functional strand is loaded into the RISC complex. The function of miRNA is depending on the complementarity of the seed region of mature miRNA to the 3'UTR of the target mRNA gene, either undergoing mRNA cleavage or translational repression. Strategies for miRNA-based therapies: improving miRNA in disease can be achieved by the following approaches: (a) Small molecule miRNA inhibitors can regulate miRNA expression at the transcriptional level. (b) Antisense oligonucleotides can bind to the target miRNA and induce degradation effect. (c) The miR-mask oligonucleotides are synthetic oligonucleotides complementary to the 3' UTR target mRNA that compete with endogenous miRNA for its target. (d) The miRNA sponges are oligonucleotide constructs with multiple complementary miRNA binding sites to the target miRNA. (e) The miRNA mimics are synthetic miRNAs which can restored the downregulated miRNA expression. (f) The AAV miRNA vectors are a group of adenovirus-associated vectors that have been inserted genes coding for miRNAs and they are used for restoring downregulated miRNA expression.

miRNA–mRNA complementarity. If there is a high degree of complementarity between the miRNA and mRNA, it will enable the Ago-catalyzed degradation of target mRNA sequences through the mRNA cleavage mechanism process. However, if there is a low degree of degree of miRNA–mRNA complementarity, a central mismatch will omit degradation and promotes the translational repression mechanism.

The exact mechanism for translational repression by miRNA is still not fully understood. However, recent studies suggest that, as the miRNA is incorporated into a RISC [3, 4], the associated protein silencing complex can either repress translational mechanisms typically associated with ribosomal translation, or induce deadenylation of the 3′ poly-A protective posttranscriptional mRNA modification, thought to be involved in repression via the mRNA 5′ terminal cap. The mechanism for mRNA degradation is mainly involved in endonucleolytic cleavage, which is facilitated by Argonaute cleavage proteins. It has been shown that when miRNAs have a high degree of sequence complementarity, then target mRNA degradation processes are facilitated through Ago protein slicer activity [2, 3]. miRNA typically binds to the 3′ untranslated region (3' UTR) in mRNA that follows the translation termination codon. The mechanism of miRNA translation inhibition requires partial sequence match, whereas the mechanism of miRNA-mediated mRNA degradation requires a near-perfect complementary match (see **Figure 1**).

4. Regulation of miRNAs

There are multiple levels of regulation of miRNA expression [5]. Those regulatory mechanisms mainly include transcriptional and post-transcriptional mechanisms, as well as effects of endogenous and exogenous compounds on the miRNA expression.

4.1 Transcriptional regulation

Similar to protein-coding genes, miRNA genes can also be regulated through transcription level. The promoters of miRNA genes are controlled by transcription factors (TFs). Many TFs regulate miRNA gene expression through positive or negative mechanism in a tissue-specific or developmental-specific manner. For instance, MYC inhibits expression of tumor suppressor miRNA-15a, which promote MYC-mediated tumorigenesis [6]. On the other hands, MYC can stimulate expression of miR-9 in neuroblastoma cells, resulting in regulation of E-cadherin and cancer metastasis [7]. It has shown that p53 enhances the expression of miR-34 and miR-107 families, which induce cell cycle arrest and apoptosis [8]. In addition to regulate by TFs, the expression of miRNA can be regulated by methylation of the promoter. Most of the miRNA promoter region has certain CpG islands. For example, promoter hypermethylation of genes such as miR-132, miR-34b/c, miR-218-1/2, and miR33b have been associated with or denote a poor prognosis of various cancers [9, 10]. In addition, the changes in DNMT1 and DNMT3b DNA methyltransferases lead to alter the miRNAs (miR-148a, miR-34b/c, miR-9 and let-7) gene promoter methylation status, resulting in regulation of their gene transcription levels [11]. Furthermore, it has reported that miR-210 is highly induced by hypoxia in various cancer cell lines [12], whose expression is not only regulated by the transcription factors hypoxia-inducible factor-1 (HIF-1), but also regulated by DNA demethylation mechanism in neural progenitor cells under both normoxia and hypoxia [12].

4.2 Post-transcriptional regulation

Post-transcriptional regulation has emerged as another important mechanism in define the miRNA expression pattern, which mainly involves the processing of the miRNA after transcription. On the post-transcriptional level, the expression of microRNAs can be downregulated due to changes in the activity of key miRNA biogenesis enzymes, such as Dicer and Drosha. Dicer and Drosha generally operate in complexes with double-stranded RBP partner (such as TRBP and DGCR8). Both the levels and activity of all of these proteins are subject to regulate the accumulation of miRNAs. For example, a decrease in TRBP leads to Dicer destabilization and pre-miRNA processing defects [9, 13]. In addition, recent studies have also demonstrated that post-translational changes in the Ago family of protein could cause significant changes in miRNA expression profiles [9, 13].

Another important contributor to miRNA levels is the stability of miRNA, which depends on the stage of development or cell type involved. It has been discovered that some proteins can bind miRNAs and affect their half-life [9, 14]. For example, HuR, a member of the ElaV family of RNA-binding proteins has been shown to suppress the inhibitory effect of miRNAs [14]. On the other hands, it has been shown that overexpression of Argonaute proteins can decelerate miRNA degradation and increase miRNA stability [9, 15].

4.3 Endogenous and xenobiotics regulation

The presence of physiological and pathological conditions have been demonstrated to regulate miRNA expression. Previous studies have shown that steroid hormones can regulate miRNA expression [16, 17]. Treatment with estradiol or tamoxifen has been shown significant changes of different miRNAs expressions in patients with breast cancer and in various breast cancer cell lines [16, 17]. In addition, corticosterone also can directly regulate miRNAs expressions [18]. Rats given chronic corticosterone showed significant behavioral disorder associated with differential regulation of 26 miRNAs in the rat prefrontal cortex [18]. Off interesting, those altered miRNAs that were modulated by corticosterone have binding sites for glucocorticoid receptor element (GRE), which were either simple, composite or tethering type within the 1-kb upstream of the transcription start site. These finding suggests that binding with GRE is a common regulatory mechanism of miRNA regulation by corticosterone.

In addition to endogenous regulation, xenobiotics can affect miRNA expression. Increasing evidence from *in vivo* and *in vitro* experiments have showed that specific carcinogen could differentially alter certain miRNAs expressions [19]. Chronic treatment with benzene in mice had showed significant changes in certain miRNAs expressions [20]. Aflatoxin B1, a genotoxic carcinogen, has been reported that it can affect the profile of miRNA expression in different animal models and cell lines [21, 22]. Therefore, miRNAs can serve as biomarkers of toxicity of carcinogen agents and may be useful for early cancer diagnosis. Furthermore, harmful life styles such as alcohol consumption and tobacco smoking can impair miRNAs expressions [23, 24]. Cigarette smoking can change microRNA profile in many human organs and induces the change of plasma miRNA expression profiles in healthy subjects [25, 26]. It has been reported that 24 miRNAs were up-regulated and 11 miRNAs were down-regulated in plasma from smokers [26]. In addition, the serum miRNA profiles in nonsmokers, smokers, and lung-cancer patients were significantly different [24].

5. Clinical implication of miRNAs

MicroRNAs are becoming well recognized as their expression levels are changed in different diseases such as cancer, liver disease, coronary heart ischemic disease, and metabolic disease. Some miRNAs are increased, whereas others are decreased in a specific disease, creating a signature miRNA pattern that could serve as a biomarker or molecular therapeutic target for a particular disease. For example, in the case of cancers, the overexpressed miRNAs are commonly considered as oncogenes. On the other hand, some of the miRNAs are expressed very low levels in certain cancerous cells and usually prevent tumor development. These groups of miRNAs are called as tumor suppressor miRNAs. Let-7 is one of these tumor suppressor miRNAs [27]. The miRNAs have remarkable potential in the clinical arena because they can be detected in the blood, serum, tissues (fresh and formalin-fixed paraffin-embedded), and fine-needle aspirate specimens. Recently, novel in situ hybridization techniques have been described to detect miRNAs in tissues, which enables direct miRNA and histomorphologic correlation [28]. The clinical implications of miRNA use in medicine are present in both diagnostic and therapeutic approaches. In miRNA-based diagnostics, miRNA expression profiling has been evaluated as a reliable diagnostic biomarker for differentiating between normal and tumor specimens [29, 30]. Ali et al. have reported that the expression of let-7c, let-7f, and miR-200c were significantly decreased in pancreas cancer patients whereas miR-486-5p and miR-451 were significantly increased in those patients compared with the normal people, which suggests that these miRNAs can be served as signature biomarkers for pancreas cancer [30]. Additionally, circulating miRNAs can be employed in diagnostic strategies to detect for alterations associated with either disorder affliction or treatment response. In the miRNA-based therapeutics, the miRNA expression is altered in different diseases and it is now feasible to correct miRNA expression by injecting miRNAs similar to the use of antisense mRNAs and RNAi. For example, because the activation of onco-miRNA genes could cause development of cancer, artificial antisense miRNAs could be synthesized and used to inhibit their targeted miRNAs to treat or prevent the cancer.

6. miRNA therapeutics: strategies

There are at least two main strategies to target miRNA expression for prevention and potential treatment of disease. The first strategies is the use of oligonucleotides or virus-based constructs to either directly block the expression of a disease-associated signature miRNA or to directly substitute for the loss of expression of the miRNA. The second strategies is indirectly employing drugs to alter miRNA expression by targeting their transcription and processing. Blocking miRNA expression can be achieved by the use of antisense oligonucleotides, miRNA sponges, miRNA-mask and small RNA inhibitors. Restoring downregulated miRNA expression can be achieved by using synthetic miRNA (miRNA mimic) or by inserting genes coding for miRNA into viral constructs. At the transcriptional level, small-molecule miRNA inhibitors can be employed to prevent the transitions from DNA transcript to pri-miRNA and pre-miRNA. Antisense oligonucleotides can be employed at the mature miRNA level to induce degradation or revert the mature miRNA into a duplex form with the antisense oligonucleotide. At the functional level, miRNA masks can bind complementarily to the 3' UTR region of target mRNA, competing for bindings with endogenous miRNAs for the specific target. miRNA sponges can be employed to bind target miRNA via complementary mRNA binding sites, decreasing expression levels of target miRNAs (see **Figure 1**).

6.1 Antisense oligonucleotides (AMO)

Antisense inhibition of miRNA function has been an important tool for uncovering miRNA biology and potential therapeutics [31]. Synthetic oligonucleotides can be used therapeutically when miRNA dysregulation contributes to pathophysiology. These oligonucleotides are known as anti-miRNA oligonucleotides (miRNA inhibitors). To improve functional potency and to provide protection against nuclease degradation, they are often chemically modified [31, 32]. An ideal modification should increase binding affinity to the extent that specificity is compromised and should be non-toxic. There are four most common oligonucleotide modifications: (1) 2'-O-methyl groups, (2) phosphorothioate, (3) locked nucleic acid (LNA) anti-miRNA constructs, and (4) N,N-diethyl-4-(4-nitronaphthalen-1-ylazo)-phenylamine (ZEN).

2'-O-methyl groups are the first generation of AMOs. 2'-O-methyl modifications can help AMOs to increase nuclease resistance and facilitate binding affinities to miRNA by the addition of an O-methyl group to the 2'-C atom. Phosphorothioate, compared to the 2'-O-methyl analogs, bonds at both the 3′ and 5′ ends to prevent nuclease degradation, and a 3′ cholesterol tail to help with cell uptake [33]. These modifications help the AMO to penetrate into tissues and organs and significantly increase their half-lives in the target tissues. However, the first generation of AMOs have relative low potencies to be effective in animal model [34]. Second generation AMOs contain other modifications at the 2′ sugar position. Locked nucleic acid (LNA) modifications which are bicyclic nucleic acids that tether the 2'O to the 4'C via methylene bridge locking sugar into a 3′ endo conformation have been shown to have the best binding affinity and nuclease resistance. This group of AMO has been widely used in experimental animals [35–37]. Currently, the most advanced miRNA targeting therapy is SPC3649 (miravirsen), which is a locked nucleic acid-modified oligonucleotide antagonizing miR-122. This is the first miRNA-targeted drug to enter human clinical trials [38]. Despite LNA modifications have higher binding affinity, these modifications can lead to off-target effects which may cause toxicity *in vivo* [35]. Recently, a new compound called N,N-diethyl-4-(4-nitronaphthalen-1-ylazo)-phenylamine (ZEN), when is included at each end of the AMO, led to increased binding affinity to the miRNA and inhibited exonuclease degradation. Recent studies have shown that this group of AMOs (ZEN-AMOs) have higher potency and less toxicity than LNA-AMOs [39].

6.2 miRNA sponges

miRNA sponges are transcripts that contain multiple (typically 4–10 separated by a few nucleotides) tandem-binding sites to a miRNA of interest and are transcribed from mammalian expression vectors. The use of miRNA sponges in mammalian cells was introduced by Ebert and colleagues [40]. miRNA sponges have been found to occur naturally as long non-coding RNA in plants and animals. Synthetic miRNA sponges are usually plasmid or viral vectors which contain tandemly arrayed miRNA binding sites, separated with a small nucleotide spacer and inserted into a 3'UTR of the reporter gene driven by an RNA polymerase II promoter [40, 41]. miRNA sponges have the ability to inhibit an entire family of miRNA by using the common seed sequence, and can therefore inhibit multiple miRNAs at once. Some of the endogenous circular RNAs have been founded to function as nature miRNA sponges. For example, circRNA7 has been shown to be functions as a miRNA sponge for miRNA-7 in the mouse tissues [42]. The authors have further demonstrated that the testis-specific circRNA, sex-determining region Y (Sry), serves as a miR-138 sponge [42]. These finding suggest that circRNA functioning as a miRNA sponge to regulate miRNA expression may be a common phenomenon in human and animals.

6.3 miRNA masking

MicroRNA-masking antisense oligonucleotide technology (miR-mask) is another strategy for miRNA-based therapeutics. In contrast to miRNA sponges, miR-masks consist of single-stranded 2'-O-methyl modified antisense oligonucleotides that are fully complementary to the expected miRNA binding site in the 3'-UTR of target mRNA [43]. A miR-mask does not directly interact with its target miRNA but binds to the binding site of that miRNA in the 3' UTR of the target mRNA by fully complementary mechanism. Therefore, the miR-mask blocks the access of its target miRNA to the binding site so as to rescue its target mRNA via blocking the action of its target miRNA. miR mask is designed to be fully complementary to the target mRNA sequence of a miRNA, which suggests that the anti-miRNA action of a miR-mask is gene-specific. The strategy of miRNA masking has been used to disrupt miRNA function and involves masking the target site on target mRNA using a modified single-stranded RNA complementary to the target sequence [44, 45]. The miRNA-masking method, in which only specific mRNA is masked, may lead to more specific and safer therapeutic strategies.

6.4 Small molecule inhibitors

Several drugs may possess the ability to modulate miRNA expression, targeting signaling pathways in miRNA biogenesis, ultimate converging on the activation of transcription factors involved in the regulation of miRNA encoding genes. The first specific molecule founded to be effective for inhibition of miRNA is an azobenzene [46]. The authors have demonstrated that the azobenzene can inhibit miRNA-21 by inhibiting miRNA-21 precursor in live cells [46]. MicroRNA-21 is significantly overexpressed in many types of human cancers, thus miR-21 is a potential therapeutic target. Recently, Naro et al. [47] have reported that, using a luciferase-based reporter assay, a high-throughput screen of >300,000 compounds led to the discovery of a new aryl amide class of small-molecule miR-21 inhibitors. Their studies further found that four aryl amide derivatives were very potent and selective miR-21 inhibitors [47]. The small molecule miRNA inhibitors are currently limited by their relatively low potencies and issues with specificity to a particular miRNA, however, they are much easier to deliver and have the promise for development of therapeutics.

6.5 miRNA mimics

In addition to miRNA inhibition as a major miRNA therapeutic approach, miRNA replacement treatment with miRNA mimics should be another miRNA therapeutic approach in disease associated with decreased miRNAs expressions. Synthetic miRNA mimics can assume the regulatory role of natural miRNAs. In diseases such as cancer, some tumor suppression-related miRNAs are downregulated. Therefore, artificial double-stranded miRNA (miRNA mimic) has been introduced to inhibit cancer [48]. Recent studies have reported that miRNA-34 is a master regulator of tumor suppression and a well-defined miRNA tumor suppressor [49]. It acts on several cancer relevant cellular pathways, including the p53 and wnt/β-catenin pathways. Down-regulation of miR-34 expression has been found in many tumor types, including lung, liver, breast, and colon carcinoma, and treatment with miR-34 mimic has been shown to inhibit tumor growth and progression [49, 50]. Consequently, miR-34 mimic, the first miRNA replacement therapy, is headed to the clinic for treatment of cancer [49, 50]. Replacement of oncosuppressor miRNAs with their mimics provides an effective strategy against cancer.

6.6 Viral vectors

Viral vector administration and encoding of miRNAs have been used for various therapeutic purposes [51]. A range of viruses can be employed for these purposes, including lentiviruses, adenoviruses, and adenoassociated viruses (AAVs). Since these vectors do not integrate into the genome, they can be eliminated efficiently with minimal toxicity, yet show remarkable efficiency in transferring RNA-encoding vectors into the nucleus of mammalian cells, ensuring high expression of miRNA [51]. Previous studies have shown that systemic lentivirus delivery of miR-15a/16 reduces lymphocytic leukemia progression in a mouse model [52]. In a murine model of muscular dystrophy-associated chronic dilated cardiomyopathy [53], intraventricular delivery of AAV vectors containing miR-669a induces long-term miR-669a overexpression and significantly decreases hypertrophic remodeling, fibrosis, and cardiomyocyte apoptosis. Furthermore, it significantly reduces adverse remodeling and enhances systolic fractional shortening of the left ventricle in treated dystrophic mice, without significant detrimental consequences on skeletal muscle wastage [53]. Viral vector therapies have shown the highest efficacy for delivering miRNA into cells and organs in vitro and in vivo. However, their safety and toxicity remains a controversial issue.

7. miRNA therapeutics in disease

miRNAs are abundant in many mammalian cell types and appear to target about 60% of the genes of humans and other mammals [54]. Many miRNAs are evolutionarily conserved, which implies that they have important biological functions. However, growing evidence suggests that alteration of miRNAs expressions plays a key role in the development of disease. The signature miRNAs associated with disease and their potential therapeutics in the most common diseases are discussed in the following sections.

7.1 Therapeutic potential of microRNAs in cancer

Rapidly growing evidence supports that miRNAs play key roles in the pathogenesis of cancer and many miRNAs can function either as oncogenes or tumor suppressors [55]. MiRNAs can influence the development, progression, and metastasis of cancers [29, 30]. Their functional effect may differ depending on their expression levels. They have either an oncogenic potential or tumor-suppressor effect depending on their downstream impact on target genes and thereby controlling the biologic manifestations of cancers. The activity of a lost or down-regulated tumor suppressor miRNA can be restored by using miRNA mimics [56]. To date, there are some miRNA-based trials for treatment of cancers. For examples, miR-34 is one of the tumor suppressor miRNAs and it is significantly downregulated in many kinds of cancer [57]. Therefore, a cancer therapy synthetic miR-34 (MRX34) has been developed and has entered phase I clinical trial for liver cancer and metastasis from other cancers (NCT01829971) [57]. In lung cancer, miR-27a has been reported to be a potential targeted therapy for lung cancer [58]. MicroRNA-loaded minicells (miR-16-based mimic miRNA) are designed to counteract the loss of the miR-15 and miR-16 family and are used in clinic trials for small-cell lung cancer and mesothelioma [59]. The miR-205BP/S3 is a possible promising therapeutic modality for melanoma [60]. Let-7 is well recognized as one of the important tumor suppressors. So re-expression of the tumor-suppressor let-7 is another proposed miRNA therapeutic strategy to upregulate tumor-suppressor miRNA by exogenously transfecting with pre-let-7 that led to the inhibition of growth [27]. In addition to tumor suppressor miRNAs, some of the miRNAs can be served as oncogenes and used as therapeutic targets for cancer. For example, miR-21 is significantly overexpressed in many types of human cancers, thus miR-21 is a potential therapeutic target for a certain cancer [47].

7.2 Therapeutic potential of microRNAs in liver disease

Numerous studies have demonstrated that alterations in intracellular miRNAs correlated with various liver diseases [28, 38, 61]. In the liver, MiR-122 is one of the highly abundant miRNAs that affects various genes involved in hepatic cholesterol and lipid metabolism, thereby playing a central role in maintaining liver homeostasis [61]. Intriguingly, miR-122 is essential to the stability and propagation of hepatitis C virus (HCV) [61]. The finding of the role of miR-122 in the HCV replication process is one of the best examples of the potential targeted miRNA-based therapeutic approaches. Blocking miR-122 using antisense approaches has reduced HCV replication in animal model [61]. MiR-122 binds to two closely spaced target sites (S1 and S2) in the highly conserved 5′ untranslated region of the HCV genome, thereby forming an oligomeric miR-122–HCV complex that protects the HCV genome from nucleolytic degradation or from host innate immune responses. Recently, a LNA-miR-122, known as Miravirsen, has been introduced and demonstrated that it can decrease HCV in nonhuman primates with no side effects [62]. Furthermore, in clinical trials of Miravirsen (NCT01200420), it has shown that the use of miravirsen in patients with chronic HCV genotype 1 infection can induce dose-dependent reductions in HCV RNA levels without evidence of viral resistance [61]. This miRNA-based therapeutics might deliver promising outcomes in the setting of liver disease.

7.3 Therapeutic potential of microRNAs in heart disease

Growing evidence shows miRNAs could be a promise molecular therapeutic strategy for cardiovascular disease [63, 64]. Previous studies have demonstrated that miRNA-21 level is upregulated in activated fibroblasts of the failing heart [65]. The investigators further demonstrated in an *in vivo* study of a mouse model of pressure-overload-induced heart disease that administration of a miRNA-21 antisense construct reduces the extent of heart fibrosis and overall heart function [65]. Their findings validate miR-21 as a disease target in heart failure and establish the therapeutic efficacy of microRNA therapeutic intervention in a cardiovascular disease setting. The miR-15 family is also found to be significantly increased in cardiac diseases [66]. Knockdown of the miR-15 family with LNA-modified anti-miRNAs resulted in reduced infarct size after ischaemia-reperfusion injury [66], suggesting it could serve as a therapeutic target for the manipulation of cardiac remodeling and function in the setting of myocardial infarction.

Diastolic dysfunction is a major clinical syndrome. Gain- and loss-of-function studies in animal model have shown that genetic deletion of the cardiac-specific miR-208a prevents pathological cardiac remodeling. Furthermore, therapeutic inhibition of miR-208a by subcutaneous delivery of miR-208a antisense during hypertension-induced heart failure in rats can prevent pathological myosin switching and cardiac remodeling and improve cardiac function [67, 68]. These studies suggest that miR-208 can serve as a potent therapeutic target for the modulation of cardiac function and remodeling during heart disease progression. In addition, miRNAs also play an important role in regulation of cardiovascular angiogenesis. AntimiR-92a (MRG-110) is currently used as a Phase I clinical trial for Miragen and it could offer a potential therapeutic to accelerate the healing process and revascularization in chronic ischemic disease. MRG-110 is being developed under a license and collaboration agreement with Servier for the treatment of heart failure and other ischemic disease [www.miragen.com]. To date, there is another therapeutics miRNA (MGN-5804 which targeting miR-378) in the development phase for the treatment of cardiovascular disease.

7.4 Therapeutic potential of microRNAs in renal disease

MicroRNAs can serve as mediators and therapeutic targets in many chronic renal diseases [69].

A variety of miRNAs are specifically enriched in the renal tissue as compared with other tissues, including miR-192, miR-194, miR-204, miR-215, and miR-216 [69]. miR-192 is one of the key miRNAs which is involved in diabetic nephropathy [70]. The authors reported that, in individual biopsies, tubulointerstitial fibrosis and low estimated GFR are associated with a decrease in miR-192 expression [70].

miR-192 targets E-cadherin, resulting in fibrosis of tubular cells and development of diabetic nephropathy. These findings suggests that miR-192 mimics should potentially be used as therapeutics of diabetic nephropathy. A global expression profiling study have shown that miR-21 is one of the most highly regulated miRNAs in kidneys of mice with diabetic nephropathy [71]. It has been reported that miR-21 antagonism in vitro and in vivo in streptozotocin-induced diabetic mice decreased mesangial expansion, interstitial fibrosis, macrophage infiltration, podocyte loss, albuminuria, and fibrotic- and inflammatory gene expression, which suggests that therapeutic miR-21 silencing could ameliorate diabetic kidney disease. Indeed, in a mouse model of chronic kidney disease, treatment with antagomir against miR-21 reverses both glomerular and tubular cell damage, resulting in a decrease in renal fibrosis and prolonging the life span of the chronic kidney disease-affected mice [72].

7.5 Therapeutic potential of microRNAs in neurological disease

Some of the miRNAs are highly abundant in the nervous system, where they play key roles in developmental neurobiology. Numerous studies have shown a dysregulation of miRNAs in neurological disease [73, 74]. These alterations in miRNAs expression prior to the onset of or during the course of disease pathology raises the possibility that expressing or inhibiting specific miRNAs might ameliorate the disease process and provide an effective therapeutic strategy. For example, Alzheimer's disease (AD) is being tested for potential miRNA-based therapy [75]. It has reported that a member of the miR-15/107 superfamily, miR-16 can specifically inhibits the expression of AD biomarkers Aβ and Tau, as well as brain inflammation and oxidative stress. MicroR-16 mimics delivered into the brain of mice resulted in a reduction of AD-related genes expression in a region-dependent manner, thus supporting the potential of miR-16 as an excellent therapeutic candidate for treatment of Alzheimer's disease. Similar to the changes of miRNAs in Alzheimer's disease, numerous miRNAs in human and animal models are also reported to be dysregulated in Parkinson's disease [76]. Some of these dysregulated miRNAs have been suggested to be potential therapeutic targets for Parkinson's disease. For example, Cho et al. had suggested that overexpression of miR-205 by miR-205 mimic could provide a potential therapeutic strategy to suppress the abnormal upregulation of LRRK2 protein in Parkinson's disease [77]. In addition, it has been reported that early downregulation of miR-34b/c in Parkinson's disease triggers downstream transcriptome alterations underlying mitochondrial dysfunction and oxidative stress, which ultimately compromise cell viability [78]. Therefore, upregulation of miR-34b/c may be an applicable therapeutic strategy for Parkinson's disease.

8. Future prospects

As the miRNA field dramatically grows, a better understanding of miRNA biogenesis and path-physiologic function will help to develop miRNA-based therapies. In addition, it is well known that a specific miRNA could target multiple genes and affect different organs in the same time. Therefore, research efforts should try to maximize the benefit of target diversity and prevent off-target effects. To achieve this goal, improvement of the chemical design of miRNA antisense and mimics and developing novel delivery systems are very important to ensure that the desired miRNA concentrations are achieved in organs and the targets are specifically regulated.

The use of synthetic miRNAs holds great promise as a new class of potential therapeutic agents by silencing the gene(s) of interest. Applicable to a wide variety of human diseases such as cancer, viral infections, genetic disorders, and cardiovascular disease, the attractiveness of miRNA therapeutics is their ability to target specific genes of interest, not always possible with small molecules or protein-based drugs. When designing drugs for therapeutic use, RNA sequence must be carefully designed to avoid undesired effects and immune responses in the body. The care into making a safe and relevant delivery system for miRNA-based therapies must also balance considerations of target tissue and cell delivery, cellular uptake, and nuclease degradation of the molecule.

Although a considerable number of clinical trials involving miRNA therapeutics have been conducted over the years, not all of those miRNA therapeutics have so far moved into clinical implication. The big challenges for miRNA-based therapeutics is to identify the best miRNA candidates or miRNA targets for each type of disease. The other challenges include the optimizing the miRNA delivery vehicles that can have higher targeting specificity and stability, as well as having lower toxicities and off-target effects. Although there are still hurdles to the use of mRNA-targeting approaches for clinical applications, with the rapid expansion occurring in this field, the prospects of miRNA-based therapeutics remain promising.

9. Conclusions

Growing evidences have shown that miRNAs play a key role in biological function and cell homeostasis. If the miRNAs are dysregulated, they lead to the development of many disease phenotypes. The miRNAs have immense potential in the clinical arena because they can be detected in the blood, serum, tissues, and fine-needle aspirate specimens. In addition, the discovery of miRNAs and their expression profile in a wide variety of diseases has led investigators to understand the key role of miRNAs as biomarkers during disease progression. Furthermore, because the miRNAs are relatively small size and they can regulate the network of target genes, they are promising targets for therapeutics. The most attractive feature of miRNA-based therapy is that a single miRNA could be useful for targeting multiple genes that are deregulated in disease, which can be further investigated through systems biology and network analysis that allows designing disease-specific personalized therapy. In summary, miRNAs are poised to provide diagnostic, prognostic, and therapeutic targets for several diseases. As the field continues to grow, miRNA-based therapeutics may develop a novel class of drugs for different diseases.

Acknowledgements

Grant support: This work was supported by National Institutes of Health (NIH) Grants NIH/HL135623, NIH/HD088039, and NIH/DA041492 (DX).

Conflict of interest

None.

Notes/Thanks/Other declarations

None.

Author details

Andrew Walayat[1], Meizi Yang[1,2] and DaLiao Xiao[1*]

1 Department of Basic Science, Center for Perinatal Biology, Loma Linda University School of Medicine, Loma Linda, California, USA

2 Department of Pharmacology, Binzhou Medical University, Yantai, China

*Address all correspondence to: dxiao@llu.edu

IntechOpen

© 2018 The Author(s). Licensee IntechOpen. This chapter is distributed under the terms of the Creative Commons Attribution License (http://creativecommons.org/licenses/by/3.0), which permits unrestricted use, distribution, and reproduction in any medium, provided the original work is properly cited.

References

[1] Lee RC, Feinbaum RL, Ambros V. The *C. elegans* heterochronic gene line-4 encodes small RNAs with antisense complementarity to lin-14. Cell. 1993;**75**(5):843-854

[2] Hammond SM. An overview of microRNAs. Advanced Drug Delivery Reviews. 2015;**87**:3-14. DOI: 10.1016/j.addr

[3] Mac Farlane LA, Murphy PR. MicroRNA: Biogenesis, function and role in cancer. Current Genomics. 2010;**11**(7):537-561

[4] Lam JKW, Chow MYT, Zhang Y, Leung SWS. SiRNA versus miRNA as therapeutics for gene silencing. Molecular Therapy-Nucleic Acids. 2015;**4**:e252

[5] Gulyaeva LF, Kushlinskiy NE. Regulatory mechanisms of microRNA expression. Journal of Translational Medicine. 2016;**14**:143

[6] Chang TC, Yu D, Lee YS, Wentzel EA, Arking DE, West KM, et al. Widespread microRNA repression by Myc contributes to tumorigenesis. Nature Genetics. 2008;**40**:43-50

[7] Ma L, Young J, Prabhala H, Pan E, Mestdagh P, Muth D, et al. miR-9, a MYC/MYCN-activated microRNA, regulates E-cadherin and cancer metastasis. Nature Cell Biology. 2010;**12**:247-256

[8] He L He X, Lim LP, de Stanchina E, Xuan Z, Liang Y, Xue W, et al. A microRNA component of the p53 tumour suppressor network. Nature. 2007;**447**:1130-1134

[9] Diederichs S, Haber DA. Dual role for argonautes in microRNA processing and posttranscriptional regulation of microRNA expression. Cell. 2007;**131**(6):1097-1108

[10] Behm-Ansmant I, Rehwinkel J, Izaurralde E. MicroRNAs silence gene expression by repressing protein expression and/or by promoting mRNA decay. Cold Spring Harbor Symposia on Quantitative Biology. 2006;**71**:523-530

[11] Han L, Witmer PD, Casey E, Valle D, Sukumar S. DNA methylation regulates microRNA expression. Cancer Biology & Therapy. 2007;**6**:1284-1288

[12] Xiong L, Wang F, Huang X, Liu Z, Zhao T, Wu L, et al. DNA demethylation regulates the expression of miR-210 in neural progenitor cells subjected to hypoxia. The FEBS Journal. 2012;**279**:4318-4326

[13] Kawahara Y. Human diseases caused by germline and somatic abnormalities in microRNA and microRNA-related genes. Congenital Anomalies (Kyoto). 2014;**54**(1):12-21

[14] Meisner NC, Filipowicz W. Properties of the regulatory RNA-binding protein HuR and its role in controlling miRNA repression. Advances in Experimental Medicine and Biology. 2011;**700**:106-123

[15] Winter J, Diederichs S. Argonaute proteins regulate microRNA stability: Increased microRNA abundance by Argonaute proteins is due to microRNA stabilization. RNA Biology. 2011;**8**(6):1149-1157

[16] Egeland NG, Lunde S, Jonsdottir K, Lende TH, Cronin-Fenton D, Gilje B, et al. The role of microRNAs as predictors of response to tamoxifen treatment in breast cancer patients. International Journal of Molecular Sciences. 2015;**16**:24243-24275

[17] Maillot G, Lacroix-Triki M, Pierredon S, Gratadou L, Schmidt S, Bénès V, et al. Widespread estrogen-dependent repression of microRNAs

involved in breast tumor cell growth. Cancer Research. 2009;**69**:8332-8340

[18] Dwivedi Y, Roy B, Lugli G, Rizavi H, Zhang H, Smalheiser NR. Chronic corticosterone-mediated dysregulation of microRNA network in prefrontal cortex of rats: Relevance to depression pathophysiology. Translational Psychiatry. 2015;**5**:e682

[19] Chen T. The role of microRNA in chemical carcinogenesis. Journal of Environmental Science and Health. Part C, Environmental Carcinogenesis & Ecotoxicology Reviews. 2010;**28**:89-124

[20] Wei H, Zhang J, Tan K, Sun R, Yin L, Pu Y. Benzene-induced aberrant miRNA expression profile in hematopoietic progenitor cells in C57BL/6 mice. International Journal of Molecular Sciences. 2015;**16**:27058-27071

[21] Liu C, Yu H, Zhang Y, Li D, Xing X, Chen L, et al. Upregulation of miR-34a-5p antagonizes AFB1-induced genotoxicity in F344 rat liver. Toxicon. 2015;**106**:46-56

[22] Marrone AK, Tryndyak V, Beland FA, Pogribny IP. MicroRNA responses to the genotoxic carcinogens aflatoxin B1 and benzo[a]pyrene in human HepaRG cells. Toxicological Sciences. 2016;**149**(2):496-502

[23] Most D, Leiter C, Blednov YA, Harris RA, Mayfield RD. Synaptic microRNAs coordinately regulate synaptic mRNAs: Perturbation by chronic alcohol consumption. Neuropsychopharmacology. 2016;**41**(2):538-548

[24] Huang J, Wu J, Li Y, Li X, Yang T, Yang Q , et al. Deregulation of serum microRNA expression is associated with cigarette smoking and lung cancer. BioMed Research International. 2014;**2014**:364316

[25] Xi S, Xu H, Shan J, Tao Y, Hong JA, Inchauste S, et al. Cigarette smoke mediates epigenetic repression of miR-487b during pulmonary carcinogenesis. The Journal of Clinical Investigation. 2013;**123**(3):1241-1261

[26] Shi B, Gao H, Zhang T, Cui Q. Analysis of plasma microRNA expression profiles revealed different cancer susceptibility in healthy young adult smokers and middle-aged smokers. Oncotarget. 2016;**7**(16):21676-21685. DOI: 10.18632/oncotarget.7866

[27] Kong D, Heath E, Chen W, Cher ML, Powell I, Heibrun L, et al. Loss of let-7 up-regulates EZH2 in prostate cancer consistent with the acquisition of cancer stem cell signatures that are attenuated by BR-DIM. PLoS One. 2012;**7**(3):e33729. DOI: 10.1371/journal

[28] Sethi S, Sethi S, Bluth MH. Clinical implication of microRNAs in molecular pathology: An update for 2018. Clinics in Laboratory Medicine. 2018;**38**(2): 237-251. DOI: 10.1016/j.cll.2018.02.003

[29] Hassan O, Ahmad A, Sethi S, Sarkar FH. Recent updates on the role of microRNAs in prostate cancer. Journal of Hematology & Oncology. 2012;**5**:9. DOI: 10.1186/1756-8722-5-9

[30] Ali S, Saleh H, Sethi S, Sarkar FH, Philip PA. MicroRNA profiling of diagnostic needle aspirates from patients with pancreatic cancer. British Journal of Cancer. 2012;**107**(8):1354-1360. DOI: 10.1038/bjc.2012.383

[31] Lennox KA, Behlke MA. Chemical modification and design of anti-miRNA oligonucleotides. Gene Therapy. 2011;**18**(12):1111-1120. DOI: 10.1038/gt.2011.100

[32] Esau CC. Inhibition of microRNA with antisense oligonucleotides. Methods. 2008;**44**(1):55-60

[33] Lennox KA, Behlke MA. A direct comparison of anti-microRNA

oligonucleotide potency. Pharmaceutical Research. 2010;**27**(9):1788-1799

[34] Krützfeldt J, Rajewsky N, Braich R, Rajeev KG, Tuschl T, Manoharan M, et al. Silencing of microRNAs *in vivo* with 'antagomirs'. Nature. 2005;**438**(7068):685-689

[35] Swayze EE, Siwkowski AM, Wancewicz EV, Migawa MT, Wyrzykiewicz TK, Hung G, et al. Antisense oligonucleotides containing locked nucleic acid improve potency but cause significant hepatotoxicity in animals. Nucleic Acids Research. 2007;**35**(2):687-700

[36] Hildebrandt-Eriksen ES, Aarup V, Persson R, Hansen HF, Munk ME, Ørum H. A locked nucleic acid oligonucleotide targeting microRNA 122 is well-tolerated in cynomolgus monkeys. Nucleic Acid Therapeutics. 2012;**22**(3):152-161

[37] Goldaracena N, Spetzler VN, Echeverri J, Kaths JM, Cherepanov V, Persson R, et al. Inducing hepatitis C virus resistance after pig liver transplantation—A proof of concept of liver graft modification using warm ex vivo perfusion. American Journal of Transplantation. 2017;**17**(4): 970-978. DOI: 10.1111/ajt.14100

[38] Baek J, Kang S, Min H. MicroRNA-targeting therapeutics for hepatitis C. Archives of Pharmacal Research. 2014;**37**(3):299-305

[39] Lennox KA, Owczarzy R, Thomas DM, Walder JA, Behlke MA. Improved performance of anti-miRNA oligonucleotides using a novel non-nucleotide modifier. Molecular Therapy: Nucleic Acids. 2013;**2**:e117

[40] Ebert MS, Sharp PA. MicroRNA sponges: Progress and possibilities. RNA. 2010;**16**(11):2043-2050. DOI: 10.1261/rna.2414110

[41] Ebert MS, Neilson JR, Sharp PA. MicroRNA sponges: Competitive inhibitors of small RNAs in mammalian cells. Nature Methods. 2007;**4**(9):721-726

[42] Hansen TB, Jensen TI, Clausen BH, Bramsen JB, Finsen B, Damgaard CK, et al. Natural RNA circles function as efficient microRNA sponges. Nature. 2013;**495**(7441):384-388

[43] Wang Z. The principles of miRNA-masking antisense oligonucleotides technology. Methods in Molecular Biology. 2011;**676**:43-49

[44] Obad S, dos Santos CO, Petri A, Heidenblad M, Broom O, Ruse C, et al. Silencing of microRNA families by seed-targeting tiny LNAs. Nature Genetics. 2011;**43**:371-378

[45] Choi WY, Giraldez AJ, Schier AF. Target protectors reveal dampening and balancing of nodal agonist and antagonist by miR-430. Science. 2007;**318**:271-274

[46] Gumireddy K, Young DD, Xiong X, Hogenesch JB, Huang Q , Deiters A. Small-molecule inhibitors of microrna miR-21 function. Angewandte Chemie (International Edition in English). 2008;**47**(39):7482-7484

[47] Naro Y, Thomas M, Stephens MD, Connelly CM, Deiters A. Aryl amide small-molecule inhibitors of microRNA miR-21 function. Bioorganic & Medicinal Chemistry Letters. 2015;**25**(21):4793-4796. DOI: 10.1016/j.bmcl.2015.07.016

[48] Winata P, Williams M, McGowan E, Nassif N, van Zandwijk N, Reid G. The analysis of novel microRNA mimic sequences in cancer cells reveals lack of specificity in stem-loop RT-qRCR-based microRNA detection. BMC Research Notes. 2017;**10**(1):600. DOI: 10.1186/s13104-017-2930-0

[49] Bader AG. miR-34—A microRNA replacement therapy is headed to the clinic. Frontiers in Genetics. 2012;**3**:120. DOI: 10.3389/fgene.2012.00120

[50] Misso G, Di Martino MT, De Rosa G, Farooqi AA, Lombardi A, Campani V, et al. Mir-34: A new weapon against cancer? Molecular Therapy: Nucleic Acids. 2014;**3**:e194. DOI: 10.1038/mtna.2014.47

[51] Geisler A, Fechner H. MicroRNA-regulated viral vectors for gene therapy. World Journal of Experimental Medicine. 2016;**6**(2):37-54. DOI: 10.5493/wjem.v6.i2.37

[52] Kasar S, Salerno E, Yuan Y, Underbayev C, Vollenweider D, Laurindo MF, et al. Systemic *in vivo* lentiviral delivery of miR-15a/16 reduces malignancy in the NZB de novo mouse model of chronic lymphocytic leukemia. Genes and Immunity. 2012;**13**(2):109-119

[53] Quattrocelli M, Crippa S, Montecchiani C, Camps J, Cornaglia AI, Boldrin L, et al. Long-term miR-669a therapy alleviates chronic dilated cardiomyopathy in dystrophic mice. Journal of the American Heart Association. 2013;**2**(4):e000284

[54] Fromm B, Billipp T, Peck LE, Johansen M, Tarver JE, King BL, et al. A uniform system for the annotation of vertebrate microRNA genes and the evolution of the human microRNAome. Annual Review of Genetics. 2015;**49**:213-242. DOI: 10.1146/annurev-genet-120213-092023

[55] Thorsen SB, Obad S, Jensen NF, et al. The therapeutic potential of microRNAs in cancer. Cancer Journal. 2012;**18**(3):275-284. DOI: 10.1097/PPO.0b013e318258b5d6

[56] Garzon R, Marcucci G, Croce CM. Targeting microRNAs in cancer: Rationale, strategies and challenges. Nature Reviews. Drug Discovery. 2010;**9**(10):775-789. DOI: 10.1038/nrd3179

[57] Beg MS, Brenner AJ, Sachdev J, Borad M, Kang YK, Stoudemire J, et al. Phase I study of MRX34, a liposomal miR-34a mimic, administered twice weekly in patients with advanced solid tumors. Investigational New Drugs. 2017;**35**(2):180-188. DOI: 10.1007/s10637-01600407-y

[58] Acunzo M, Romano G, Palmieri D, Lagana A, Garofalo M, Balatti V, et al. Cross-talk between MET and EGFR in non-small cell lung cancer involves miR-27a and Sprouty2. Proceedings of the National Academy of Sciences of the United States of America. 2013;**110**(21):8573-8578. DOI: 10.1073/pnas.1302107110

[59] van Zandwilk H, Pavlakis N, Kao SC, Linton A, Boyer MJ, Clarke S. Safety and activity of microRNA-loaded minicells in patients with recurrent malignant pleural mesothelioma: A first-in-man, phase 1, open-label, dose-escalation study. The Lancet Oncology. 2017;**18**:1386-1396. DOI: 10.1016/S1470-2045(17)30621-6

[60] Noguchi S, Iwasaki J, Kumazaki M, Mori T, Maruo K, Sakai H, et al. Chemically modified synthetic microRNA-205 inhibits the growth of melanoma cells in vitro and in vivo. Molecular Therapy. 2013;**21**(6):1204-1211. DOI: 10.1038/mt.2013.70

[61] Janssen HL, Reesink HW, Lawitz EJ, Zeuzem S, Rodriguez-Torres M, Patel K, et al. Treatment of HCV infection by targeting microRNA. The New England Journal of Medicine. 2013;**368**(18):1685-1694. DOI: 10.1056/NEJMoa1209026

[62] Lanford RE, Hildebrandt-Eriksen ES, Petri A, Persson R, Lindow M, Munk ME, et al. Therapeutic silencing of microRNA-122 in primates with

chronic hepatitis C virus infection. Science. 2010;**327**(5962):198-201

[63] Samanta S, Balasubramanian S, Rajasingh S, Patel U, Dhanasekaran A, Dawn B. MicroRNA: A new therapeutic strategy for cardiovascular diseases. Trends in Cardiovascular Medicine. 2016;**26**:407-419. DOI: 10.1016/j.tcm.2016.02.004

[64] Kwekkeboom RFJ, Lei Z, Doevendans PA, Musters RJP, Sluijter JPG. Targeted delivery of miRNA therapeutics for cardiovascular diseases: Opportunities and challenges. Clinical Science. 2014;**127**:351-365. DOI: 1o.1042/CS20140005

[65] Thum T, Gross C, Fiedler J, Fischer T, Kissler S, Bussen M, et al. MicroRNA-21 contributes to myocardial disease by stimulating MAP kinase signaling in fibroblasts. Nature. 2008;**456**(7224):980-984. DOI: 10.1038/nature07511

[66] Hullinger TG, Montgomery RL, Seto AG, Dickinson BA, Semus HM, Lynch JM. Inhibition of miR-15 protects against cardiac ischemic injury. Circulation Research. 2012;**110**: 71-81. DOI: 10.1161/CIRCRESAHA.111.244442

[67] van Rooij E, Quiat D, Johnson BA, Sutherland LB, Qi X, Richardson JA, et al. A family of microRNAs encoded by myosin genes governs myosin expression and muscle performance. Developmental Cell. 2009;**17**:662-673

[68] Montgomery RL, Hullinger TG, Semus HM, Dickinson BA, Seto AG, Lynch JM, et al. Therapeutic inhibition of miR-208a improves cardiac function and survival during heart failure. Circulation. 2011;**124**(14):1537-1547. DOI: 10.1161/CIRCULATIONAHA.111.030932

[69] Lorenzen JM, Haller H, Thum T. MicroRNAs as mediators and therapeutic targets in chronic kidney disease. Nature Reviews. Nephrology. 2011;7:286-294

[70] Krupa A, Jenkins R, Luo DD, Lewis A, Phillips A, Fraser D. Loss of microRNA-192 promotes fibrogenesis in diabetic nephropathy. Journal of the American Society of Nephrology. 2010;**21**:438-447

[71] Kolling M, Kaucsar T, Schauerte C, Hubner A, Dettling A, Park JK, et al. Therapeutic miR-21 silencing ameliorates diabetic kidney disease in mice. Molecular Therapy. 2017;**25**(1):165-180. DOI: 10.1016/j.ymthe.2016.08.001

[72] Gomez IG, Nakagawa N, Duffield JS. MicroRNAs as novel therapeutic targets to treat kidney injury and fibrosis. American Journal of Physiology. Renal Physiology. 2016;**310**:F931-F944

[73] Hébert SS, Horré K, Nicolaï L, Papadopoulou AS, Mandemakers W, Silahtaroglu AN, et al. Loss of microRNA cluster miR-29a/b-1 in sporadic Alzheimer's disease correlates with increased BACE1/beta-secretase expression. Proceedings of the National Academy of Sciences of the United States of America. 2008;**105**(17):6415-6420

[74] Johnson R, Zuccato C, Belyaev ND, Guest DJ, Cattaneo E, Buckley NJ. A microRNA-based gene dysregulation pathway in Huntington's disease. Neurobiology of Disease. 2008;**29**(3):438-445

[75] Parsi S, Smith PY, Goupil C, Dorval V, Hebert SS. Preclinical evaluation of miR-15/107 family members as multifactorial drug targets for Alzheimer's disease. Molecular Therapy: Nucleic Acids. 2015;**4**:e256. DOI: 10.1038/mtna.2015.33

[76] Martinez B, Peplow PV. MicroRNAs in Parkinson's disease and emerging

therapeutic targets. Neural Regeneration Research. 2017;**12**:1945-1959

[77] Cho HJ, Liu G, Jin SM, Parisiadou L, Xie C, Yu J, et al. MicroRNA-205 regulates the expression of Parkinson's disease-related leucine-rich repeat kinase 2 protein. Human Molecular Genetics. 2013;**22**:608-620

[78] Miñones-Moyano E, Porta S, Escaramís G, Rabionet R, Iraola S, Kagerbauer B, et al. MicroRNA profiling of Parkinson's disease brains identifies early downregulation of miR-34b/c which modulate mitochondrial function. Human Molecular Genetics. 2001;**20**:3067-3078